DISEASES AND DISORDERS OF CATTLE

ROGER W BLOWEY

BSc BVSc MRCVS
Wood Veterinary Group
Gloucester
England

A DAVID WEAVER

BSc Dr med vet PhD FRCVS
Department of Veterinary Medicine and Surgery
College of Veterinary Medicine
University of Missouri-Columbia
Columbia
Missouri
USA

With a Foreword by
Douglas Blood

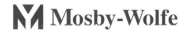 Mosby-Wolfe

London Baltimore Barcelona Bogotá Boston Buenos Aires Carlsbad, CA Chicago Madrid Mexico City Milan Naples, FL New York
Philadelphia St. Louis Seoul Singapore Sydney Taipei Tokyo Toronto Wiesbaden

Copyright © R W Blowey and A D Weaver, 1991
Published by Wolfe Publishing Ltd, 1991
Reprinted 1997 by Mosby–Wolfe, an imprint of Times Mirror International Publishers Ltd
Printed in Spain by Grafos SA, Barcelona

ISBN 0 7234 1597 8

For full details of all Times Mirror International Publishers Limited titles please write to Times Mirror International Publishers Limited, Lynton House, 7–12 Tavistock Square, London WC1H 9LB, England.

A CIP catalogue record for this book is available from the British Library.

Contents

Foreword

Textbooks dealing with diseases of cattle have never been good sources of photographic illustrations. They have either omitted pictures altogether or included a collection of disastrous black and white photographs of very poor quality. When I heard that Wolfe were to supplement their excellent collection of colour atlases with one dealing with cattle diseases it was obvious that future books would not feel obliged to add to the existing pictorial indiscretions. This was especially so because my colleagues Roger Blowey in the U.K. and David Weaver in the U.S.A. were bovine clinicians of long and wide experience covering two continents.

The need for these illustrations is obvious. For students at all stages in their careers, good colour pictures can add enormously to their understanding and ability to recognise individual diseases. In recognition of this, most clinical teachers accumulate their own colour transparencies. On several occasions I have looked at my own collection with a speculative eye, but discarded the idea because, like most amateur photographs, they lack the quality that an atlas demands. Most importantly they must illustrate the clinical signs by which the particular disease is recognised. There is no point in a photograph of a thin cow with its head hung down to illustrate tuberculosis, acetonaemia or cobalt deficiency, or a dozen other diseases. What are needed are photographs containing explicit details of specific signs. The photographs also need to be models of photographic artistry, well lit, well composed, with good contrast. Roger Blowey and David Weaver have, for their part, ensured that the photographs are truly illustrative and educational, and that the captions point up the salient features of each illustration in the minimum number of well chosen words.

Many authors, including myself, must have contemplated this task because of its potentially enormous value to veterinary medicine. I congratulate Wolfe and the authors on their courage and perseverance in going ahead and getting it done.

Douglas C. Blood
Professor Emeritus
School of Veterinary Science
University of Melbourne

Preface

For centuries cattle have been the major species for meat and milk production, and in some countries they also serve an additional role as draught animals. Disease, leading to suboptimal production or death, can have a major economic effect on a community reliant on cattle. This atlas attempts to illustrate the clinical features of over 360 conditions. These range from minor problems, such as necrosis caused by tail bands (used for identification purposes), to major infectious diseases, such as foot-and-mouth and rinderpest, which can wreak havoc when introduced into countries and areas previously free of infection. In endemic areas, which all too often include developing countries short of natural resources, they can be a constant source of serious economic loss.

To emphasise the worldwide scope of cattle diseases, we have deliberately sought illustrations from many countries. Over one hundred contributors (acknowledged elsewhere) have graphically given this atlas a truly global perspective. Examples come from all five continents: the Americas, Africa, Asia, Europe, and Australasia.

Wherever possible, we have tried to illustrate characteristic features of disorders. This has involved the use of a substantial number of internal views of animals. Thus, while the integument chapter comprises almost exclusively external views, the respiratory and circulatory sections inevitably contain much more gross pathology. Where single characteristic features do not exist, we have attempted to show typically severe examples of the conditions. Some are difficult to demonstrate in still photography, and this is particularly true of nervous diseases, where the text has been expanded to include behavioural changes.

Each chapter has a brief introductory outline followed, where appropriate, by a grouping of related conditions. No attempt has been made to consider treatment or management of specific conditions, as the atlas is designed to be used alongside standard textbooks. The major emphasis is on the diagnosis and differential diagnosis of conditions, based on visual examination. This aim has been followed with the likely readership in mind: the veterinarian in practice or government service, veterinary students, livestock producers, and agricultural and science students.

We have deliberately excluded microscopic, histopathological and cytological illustrations, since space precludes the large range of illustrations that would have been necessary. Our purpose is to make the atlas comprehensive over the range of international diseases in terms of gross features. In presenting this first attempt at a comprehensive world atlas of cattle diseases, the authors appreciate that some areas may not be covered sufficiently. We welcome suggestions and submissions for improvements to a second edition. We hope that the use of this book will aid and improve the diagnosis of cattle diseases, so permitting the earlier application of appropriate treatment and control measures. We would feel amply rewarded if the atlas helped to reduce both the substantial economic losses and the unnecessary pain and discomfort endured by cattle affected by the many health problems that hinder optimal productivity.

Roger W. Blowey
Gloucester, England

A. David Weaver
Columbia, Missouri, USA

Acknowledgements

We are very grateful to our many colleagues throughout the world who have generously allowed us access to, and use of, their transparencies and have often spent a considerable amount of time selecting them for us. Their help has been invaluable.

Material was supplied by:

Mr J.R.D. Allison, Beechams Animal Health, Brentford, England, 428, 429, 611. Prof S. van Amstel, University of Pretoria, South Africa, 650, 651. Dr E.C. Anderson, Animal Virus Research Institute, Pirbright, England, 635-640. Dr A.H. Andrews, Royal Veterinary College, England, 87, 178, 458. Prof J. Armour, Glasgow University Veterinary Hospital, Scotland, 149. Mr I.D. Baker, Aylesbury, England, 218, 383, 545. Dr K.C. Barnett, Animal Health Trust, Newmarket, England, 420, 421. Dr A. Bridi, MSD Research Laboratories, Sao Paulo, Brazil, 106, 108, 110, 111. Dr W.F. Cates, Western College of Veterinary Medicine, Canada, 528. Clinic for Diseases of Cattle, Tierärztliche Hochschule Hannover, Germany (Prof M. Stöber), 471, 479-481. Clinic of Gynaecology and Obstetrics of Cattle, Tierärztliche Hochschule Hannover, Germany (Prof E. Grunert), 535. Dr J.E. Collins, University of Minnesota, USA, 41, 42. Dr K. Collins, University of Missouri-Columbia, USA, 449. Dr B.S. Cooper, Massey University, New Zealand, 434. Dr R.P. Cowart, University of Missouri-Columbia, USA, 1. Dr V. Cox, University of Minnesota, USA, 333, 335, 385. Dr R. Crandell, San Dimas Animal Hospital, Calfornia, USA, 482. Mr M.P. Cranwell, MAFF VI Centre, Exeter, England, 703. C. Daborn, CTVM, Edinburgh, Scotland, 240-242. Dr J.S.E. David, University of Bristol, England, 337, 529, 530, 532-534, 536, 537, 539-542. Drs J. DeBont and J. Vercruysse, Rijksuniversiteit te Gent, Belgium, 212. Prof A. De Moor, Rijksuniversiteit te Gent, Belgium, 13, 352, 396. Prof J. Döbereiner and Dr C.H. Tokarnia, Embrapa-UAPNPSA, Rio de Janeiro, Brazil, 67, 158, 159, 407, 408, 412, 416, 477, 689, 702, 711, 712, 714, 715, 721. Dr A.I. Donaldson, Animal Virus Research Institute, Pirbright, England, 630-633. Dr J. van Donkersgoed, Western College of Veterinary Medicine, Canada, 425. Prof G.B. Edwards, University of Liverpool, England, 190. Dept. of Entomology, Onderstepoort, VRI, South Africa (A. Shakespeare), 93, 94. Dept. of Helminthology, Onderstepoort, VRI, South Africa (A. Shakespeare), 210, 211. Dept. of Surgery, Veterinary Faculty, Brno, Czechoslovakia, 375. Dept. of Veterinary Pathology, University of Missouri-Columbia, USA, 19, 20, 45, 55, 142, 171, 177, 184, 205, 225, 231, 244, 248, 361, 470, 473, 474, 494, 495, 518, 524, 645, 704. Prof Fan Pu, Jiangxi Agricultural University, People's Republic of China, 730. Prof J. Ferguson, Western College of Veterinary Medicine, Canada, 367, 386. Mr A.B. Forbes, MSD Agvet, Hoddesdon, England, 91, 92, 104. Mr J. Gallagher, MAFF VI Centre, Exeter, England, 130, 137, 138, 243, 398, 403, 410, 411, 413, 414, 463, 464, 564, 580, 683. Dr J.H. Geurink, Centre for Agrobiological Research, Wageningen, Netherlands, 724, 725. Dr E. Paul Gibbs, University of Florida, USA. 131, 132, 140, 221, 224, 226-228, 237, 482, 597-600, 602-604. Mr P.A. Gilbert-Green, Harare, Zimbabwe, 648. Dr H. Gosser, University of Missouri-Columbia, USA. 214, 215, 707-709. Dr W.T.R. Grimshaw, Pfizer Central Research, Sandwich, England, 24, 163, 207, 254, 492, 693, 694, 698, 699, 701. Dr S.C. Groom, Alberta Agriculture, Canada, 475. Dr Jon Gudmundson, Western College of Veterinary Medicine, Canada, 161, 251, 253, 255, 406, 472. Mr S.D. Gunn, Penmellyn Veterinary Group, St Columb, England, 487. Dr S.K. Hargreaves, Director of Veterinary Services, Harare, Zimbabwe, 629, 663, 665, 682, 710. Prof M. Hataya, Tokyo, Japan, 9, 321. Prof C.F.B. Hofmeyr, Pretoria, South Africa, 506, 523. Mr A.R. Hopkins, Tiverton, England, 508, 573. Dr L.F. James, USDA Agricultural Research Service, Logan, USA, 716. Mr P.G.H. Jones, MSD, Hoddesdon, England, 150, 245. Prof Peter Jubb, University of Melbourne, Australia, 409. Prof R. Kahrs, University of Missouri-Columbia, USA, 131, 132, 221, 224, 226, 227. Mr J.M. Kelly, University of Edinburgh, Scotland, 456. Mr D.C. Knottenbelt, University of Liverpool, England, 462, 521. Dr R. Kuiper, State University of Utrecht, Netherlands, 101,

188, 189. Dr A. Lange, University of Pretoria, South Africa, 669, 672. Dr H. Leipold, Kansas State University, USA 18. Dr L. Logan-Henfrey, International Laboratory for Research on Animal Diseases, Kenya, 666-668, 680, 681. Mrs A. MacKellar, Tavistock, England, 655-658, 660. MAFTech Ruakura Agricultural Centre, New Zealand (B.L. Smith), 719, 720. Mr K. Markham, Langport, England, 3, 15, 58, 79, 208, 284, 644. Dr M. McLellan, University of Queensland, Australia, 454, 661, 664. Mrs M.F. McLoughlin, Veterinary Research Laboratories, Belfast, N. Ireland, 690. Dr C.A. Mebus, APHIS Plum Island Animal Disease Center, USA, 649. Medizinische Tierklinik II, Universität München, Germany (Prof G. Dirksen), 713. Dr M. Miller, University of Missouri-Columbia, USA, 152, 213, 216, 232, 239, 249. Dr A. Morrow, CTVM, Edinburgh, Scotland, 97-99, 103, 652. Dr C. Mortellaro, University of Milan, Italy, 306. Dr D.R. Nawathe, University of Maiduguri, Nigeria, 634. Dr S. Nelson, University of Missouri-Columbia, USA, 47. Dr S. Nicholson, Louisiana State University, USA, 729. Dr P.S. Niehaus, Jerome, USA, 359. Dr J.K. O'Brien, University of Bristol, England, 21, 118, 144, 223, 273, 311, 330, 423, 465. Dr G. Odiawo, University of Zimbabwe, Zimbabwe, 673-675. Dr O.E. Olsen, South Dakota State University, USA, 717. Mr D.J. O'Rourke, Pitman-Moore, Uxbridge, England, 246. Prof A.L. Parodi, École Nationale Vétérinaire d'Alfort, France, 404, 405. Prof H. Pearson, University of Bristol, England, 8, 10, 198, 202, 259, 499, 513-515, 519, 520, 569, 692. Dr Lyall Petrie, Western College of Veterinary Medicine, Canada, 63, 90, 143, 180, 503, 504. Mr P.J.N. Pinsent, University of Bristol, England, 50, 64, 194, 351, 700. Prof G.H. Rautenbach, MEDUNSA, South Africa, 646, 722. Dr C.S. Ribble, Western College of Veterinary Medicine, Canada, 7. Dr A.

Richardson, Harrogate, England, 5. Dr J.M. Rutter, CVL, Weybridge, England, 230. Dr D.W. Scott, New York State College of Veterinary Medicine, USA, 81, 83. Dr A. Shakespeare, Onderstepoort, South Africa, 93, 94, 95, 210, 211. Dr M. Shearn, Institute for Animal Health, Compton, England, 608, 609, 612, 614. Dr J.L. Shupe, Utah State University, USA. 718, 727, 728. Dr Marian Smart, Western College of Veterinary Medicine, Canada, 415. Dr D.F. Smith, New York College of Veterinary Medicine, USA, 120. Mr S.E.G. Smith, Hoechst UK Ltd, Milton Keynes, England, 39, 247, 490. Mr T.K. Stephens, Frome, England, 6, 65, 72, 77, 78, 133, 135, 146, 203, 236, 252, 278, 283, 288, 294, 295, 298, 322, 342, 389, 424, 431, 435, 436, 447, 543, 578, 584, 588, 607, 615. Dr S.M. Taylor, Veterinary Research Laboratories, Belfast, N. Ireland, 148, 209. Prof H.M. Terblanche, MEDUNSA, South Africa, 261, 516, 568. Dr E. Teuscher, Lausanne, Switzerland, 676-679. Mr I. Thomas, Llandeilo, Wales, 476. Dr E. Toussaint Raven, State University of Utrecht, Netherlands, 307. Mr S. Tupper, Holstein Friesian Society, Rickmansworth, England, 289, 290. Mr N. Twiddy, MAFF VI Centre, Lincoln, England, 397, 452, 485. Dr C.B. Usher, MSD Research Laboratories, Sao Paulo, Brazil, 107, 109. Dr W.M. Wass, Iowa State University, USA, 26, 27. Mr C.A. Watson, MAFF VI Centre, Bristol, England, 25. Mr C.L. Watson, Gloucester, England, 433. Dr D.G. White, Royal Veterinary College, England, 16, 100, 264, 346, 347, 659, 695. Dr R. Whitlock, University of Pennsylvania, USA, 2, 66, 102, 154, 155, 179, 183, 191, 217, 326, 334, 345, 348, 360, 368-370, 374, 402, 442, 486, 685, 687, 688, 697. Dr W.A. Wolff, University of Missouri-Columbia, USA, 250, 256, 627. Dr Mark Zweyemann, University of Florida, USA, 597, 598.

Illustration numbers 33, 40, 327, 457, 505, 582 and 613 have been published previously by The Farming Press Ltd in *A Veterinary Book for Dairy Farmers*; 21, 456, 513, 515 and others by the *Veterinary Record* and *In Practice;* 427 and 475 by the *Canadian Veterinary Journal*; 724 and 725 by Stikstof, Netherlands; 506 and 523 by Iowa State Press; 602 and 603 by W.B. Saunders and 513 and 514 by Baillière Tindall in *Veterinary Reproduction and Obstetrics,* 6th edn, 1989.

From the University of Missouri-Columbia, gratitude is due to many clinical and pathological colleagues for useful advice and their readiness to be slide-quizzed. Glenda Allen and Vickie Robinson of Steno services and Debbie Becker of the College of Veterinary Medicine are thanked for secretarial help, and Don Connor and Howard Wilson for photography, together with A. Conibear of Bristol University Veterinary Field Station. From the UK, we would like to thank once again the many farmers of Gloucestershire who had to pause, often at the most inconvenient times, while photographs were taken; Catherine Girdler for extensive secretarial help, and Norma Blowey for endless patience, food and coffee during never-ending slide-selection sessions. We are both indebted to Professor Douglas Blood for his encouragement and for writing the Foreword.

1 Congenital disorders

Introduction

Congenital defects or diseases are abnormalities of structure or function that are present at birth. Not all congenital defects are caused by genetic factors. Some are due to environmental agents acting as teratogens. Examples include toxic plants (e.g., *Lupinus* species in crooked calf disease), prenatal viral infections (e.g., bovine virus diarrhoea (BVD) resulting in cerebellar hypoplasia and hydrocephalus), and mineral deficiencies in dams of affected calves (e.g., manganese causing skeletal abnormalities).

Hereditary bovine defects are pathologically determined by mutant genes or chromosomal aberrations. Genetic defects are classified as lethal, sublethal and subvital (including compatibility with life). Although typically occurring once or twice in every 500 births, a massive range of congenital disorders affecting different body systems has been identified in cattle, primarily as a result of records kept by artificial insemination (AI) organisations and breed societies. Economic losses are low overall, but abnormalities may cause considerable financial loss to individual pedigree breeders. Most congenital abnormalities are

evident on external examination. About half of all calves with congenital defects are stillborn. Many of these stillbirths have no clearly established cause.

Examples of congenital defects are given by affected system. Some are single skeletal defects, others are systemic skeletal disorders such as chondrodysplasia. Certain congenital central nervous system (CNS) disorders may not manifest their first clinical effects until weeks or months after birth, e.g., cerebellar hypoplasia and spastic paresis respectively.

If several neonatal calves have similar defects, an epidemiological investigation is warranted. This should include the history of the dams (their nutrition and diseases, any drug therapy during gestation, and any movement of the dams onto premises with possible teratogens), and any possible relationship of season, newly introduced stock, as well as pedigree analysis.

Congenital ocular defects are considered elsewhere (Chapter 8), as are umbilical hernia (**34**), cryptorchidism (**509**), pseudohermaphroditism (**506**) and cerebellar hypoplasia (**131**).

Cleft lip ('harelip', cheilognathoschisis); cleft palate (palatoschisis)

A failure of midline fusion during foetal development can lead to defects that affect different parts of the skeleton. Two obvious cranial abnormalities are illustrated here. A cleft lip in a young Shorthorn calf is shown in **1**, in which a deep groove extends obliquely across the upper lip, nasolabial plate and jaw, involving not only skin but also bone (maxilla). This calf had extreme difficulty in sucking milk from the dam without considerable loss through regurgitation.

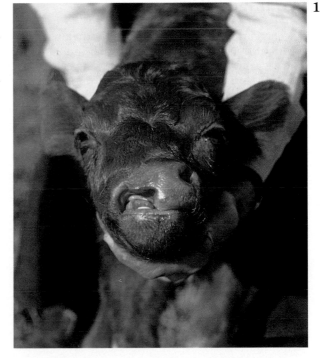

1

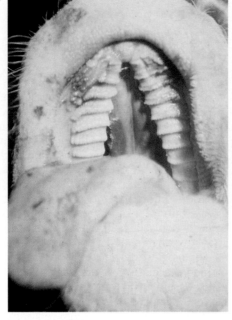

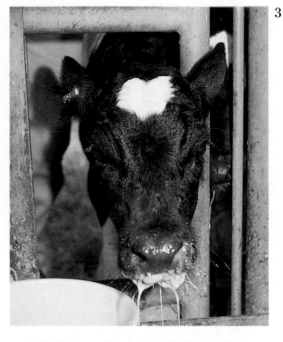

A congenital fissure or split of varying width is seen occasionally in the hard palate, or in both the hard and soft palates of neonatal calves (**2**). The major presenting sign is nasal regurgitation, as seen in the Friesian calf (**3**). An aspiration pneumonia often develops early in life from inhalation of milk, and in some while they are still nursing. Cleft palate is often associated with other congenital defects, particularly arthrogryposis. The Holstein calf (**2**) was a 'bulldog' (see **5**). Other midline defects include spina bifida (**15**) and ventricular septal defect (**24**).

Meningocoele

The large, red, fluid-filled sac (**4**) is the meninges protruding through a midline cleft in the frontal bones. The sac contains cerebrospinal fluid. The calf, a four-day-old Hereford crossbred bull, was otherwise healthy. An inherited defect was unlikely in this case. (See also **15**)

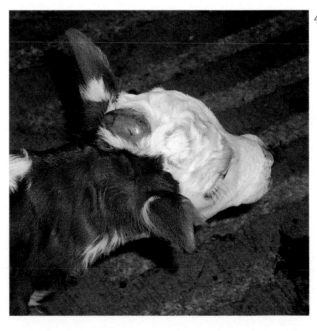

Achondroplastic dwarfism ('bulldog calf')

The Hereford calf (**5**) demonstrates a brachycephalic dwarfism. The head is short and abnormally broad, the lower jaw is overshot and the legs are very short. The abdomen was also enlarged. The calf had difficulty in standing, was dyspnoeic as a result of the skull deformity and a cleft palate was also present.

Bulldog calves are often born dead (**6**). This Ayrshire has a large head and short legs, but also has extensive subcutaneous oedema (anasarca). Dwarfism is inherited in several breeds.

A related condition is congenital joint laxity and dwarfism (CJLD), which is a distinctive congenital anomaly in beef cattle in Canada. The newborn calf (**7**) has a crouched appearance, short legs, metacarpophalangeal hyperextension and sickle-shaped hind legs. Many calves are disproportionate dwarfs. The joints become stable within two weeks and the calves then walk normally. Other organ abnormalities are not seen.

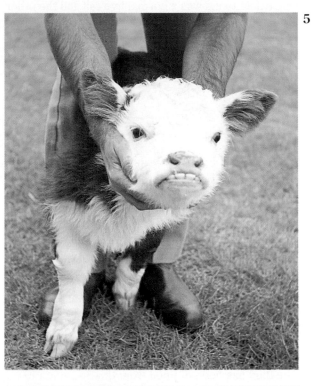

5

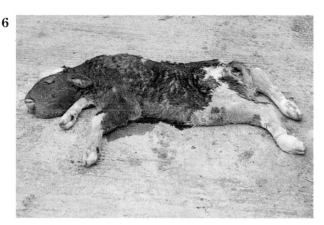

6

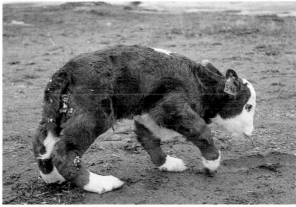

7

Schistosomus reflexus

One calf of twins was a normal live calf and the other was a schistosomus reflexus (**8**). The hindquarters are twisted towards the head, the ventral abdominal wall is open and the viscera are exposed. This anomaly usually causes dystocia.

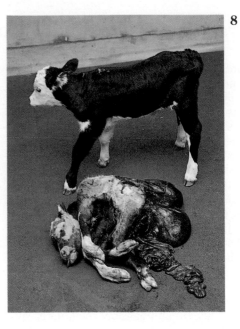

Hydranencephaly

In hydranencephaly the cerebral hemispheres are absent and their site is occupied by cerebrospinal fluid. The fluid has been drained from this specimen (**9**) after removal of the meninges. Hydranencephaly and arthrogryposis occur as a combined defect in epidemic form following certain intrauterine viral infections, e.g., Akabane virus.

Hydrocephalus

The cranium (**10**) is enlarged due to pressure from an excessive volume of cerebrospinal fluid within the ventricular system. Though usually congenital in calves, it also can occur as a rare acquired condition in adult cattle, through infection or trauma. In one form of bovine hydrocephalus there is achondroplastic dishing of the face and a foreshortened maxilla ('bulldog', see **5**).

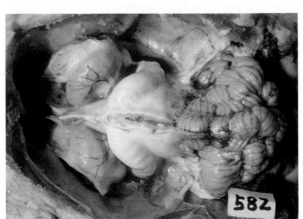

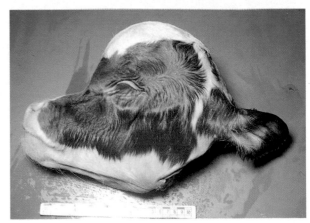

Contracted tendons

Congenital contraction of the flexor tendons in this neonatal Hereford crossbred calf (**11**) has caused excessive flexion of the carpal and fetlock joints in the forelimbs. The hind legs are placed under the body to improve weightbearing. The affected joints may be manually extended. Pectoral amyotonia is frequently present. Some forms of the condition are inherited through an autosomal recessive gene. Rarely, cases are associated with cleft palate (**2**).

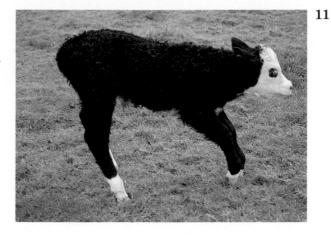

Arthrogryposis

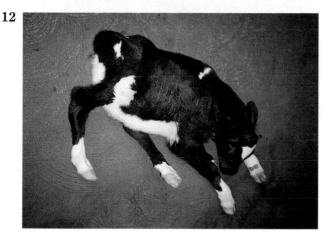

Arthrogryposis (**12**) is an extreme form of contracted tendons, in which many joints are fixed in flexion or extension (ankylosed). Frequently, two, three or all four limbs are involved in various combinations of flexion and extension. This calf has torticollis. The left foreleg is rotated about 180° (note the position of the dewclaws) and the right hind leg is sickle-shaped. Many such foetuses cause dystocia if carried to term. Some cases involve an *in utero* viral infection, e.g., Akabane virus (see p.10).

Vertebral fusion and kyphosis

Fusion of most of the cervical, thoracic and lumbar vertebrae in this two-week-old Holstein calf (**13**) was associated with a shortened neck and increased convex curvature of the spine (kyphosis). The aetiology is unknown. Kyphosis may also be an acquired condition (see **345**).

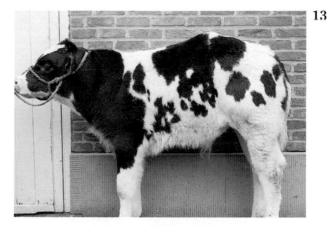

Atresia ani and hypoplastic tail

Congenital absence of the anus (**14**) is manifested clinically by an absence of faeces and the gradual development of abdominal distension. A small dimple may indicate the position of the anal sphincter. Some calves have a soft bulge from the pressure of accumulating faeces. Calves may show marked colic within three days. A fistula may develop between the rectum and urogenital tract, in this case with the pelvic urethra (see also **38**). This calf also has a 'wry tail' or hypoplastic coccyx.

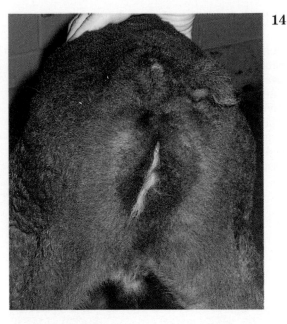

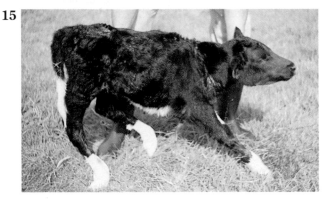

Spina bifida

Severe posterior paresis is seen in this Friesian neonate (**15**). The red, raised and circumscribed protruberance in the sacral region involves a myelomeningocoele (protrusion of both cord and meninges). The congenital defect is due to an absence of the dorsal portion of the spine (compare **4**).

Hypospadia

In this rare, male congenital anomaly, the urethra opens onto the perineum below the anus (**16**). The rudimentary penis is seen as a pink groove. There is urine staining of the inguinal region below.

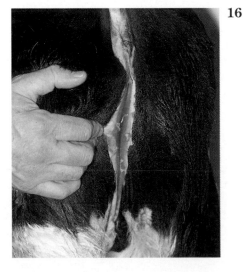

Segmental jejunal aplasia

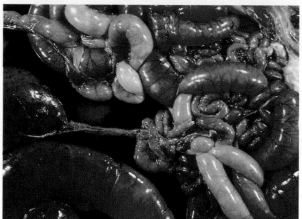

To the right, the proximal jejunum is grossly distended with fluid, as the calf (**17**), a one-week-old Charbray, initially suckled normally. The distal jejunum is empty owing to jejunal aplasia and stenosis. Meconium was present in the large intestine. The calf had developed progressive abdominal distension from four days old.

Other cases of intestinal aplasia can involve the ileum, colon and rectum, producing similar signs. However, proximal intestinal obstruction tends to produce a more acute and rapidly progressive condition. In some cases the intestine opens into the abdominal cavity, causing peritonitis and death within 48 hours. *Differential diagnosis:* mesenteric torsion (**202**) and intussusception (**203**).

Syndactyly ('mule foot')

The claws of both forelegs of this Holstein bull calf (**18**) arc fuscd. This congenital defect is due to homozygosity of a simple autosomal recessive gene with incomplete penetrance. It is the most common inherited skeletal defect of US Holstein cattle, but also occurs in several other breeds. One or more limbs may be affected.

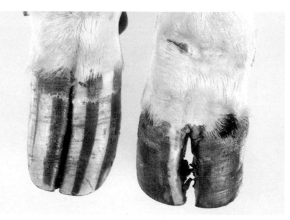

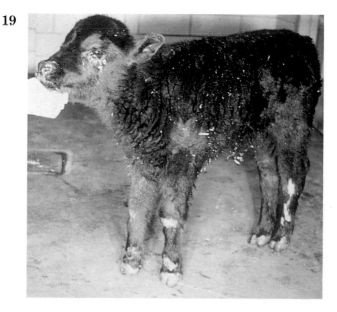

Epitheliogenesis imperfecta

Epitheliogenesis imperfecta is a congenital absence of the skin, in this case (**19**) involving thc digital horn. It is a rare sublethal defect in various breeds, inherited as a simple autosomal recessive gene. Large epithelial defects can involve the distal parts of the limbs as well as the muzzle, tongue and hard palate. Bleeding and secondary infection lead to septicaemia and early death.

Hypotrichosis

In one form of this inherited condition, viable hypotrichosis, the coat hair is thin, wavy and silky (**20**). The wrinkled skin (A) is only 2–3 cells thick. The calf has several areas of abraded skin including the carpus and the elbow. A simple autosomal recessive trait is recorded in Herefords. In another form, lethal hypotrichosis, calves, usually hairless, are born dead or die shortly afterwards.

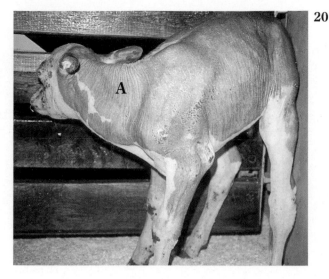

Parakeratosis (adema disease, lethal trait A46)

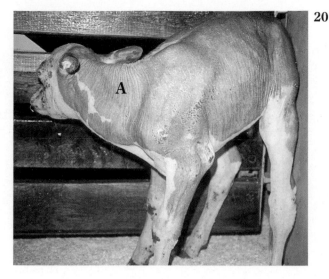

21

Parakeratosis is an inherited defect, which in Friesian cattle is associated with a poor intestinal uptake of zinc. Calves eventually die unless treated. This calf (**21**) was normal at birth, but developed a generalised parakeratosis at five weeks old. The skin of the head and neck has become thickened with scales, cracks and fissures. Above the eye, the underlying surface is raw.

Baldy calf syndrome

This Hereford-cross calf (**22**) was severely depressed, with pyrexia, poor appetite, lacrimation and nasal discharge. Areas of alopecia appeared over the head and neck. A congenital disorder that is mainly seen in Holsteins, most cases are destroyed owing to chronic unthriftiness. Both baldy calf syndrome and parakeratosis (**21**) respond to oral zinc supplementation.

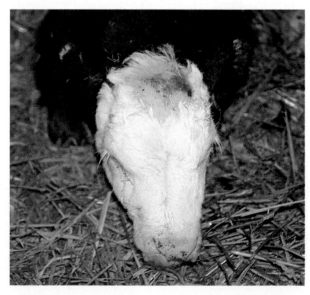

Ventricular septal defect (VSD)

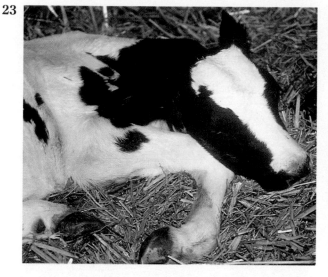

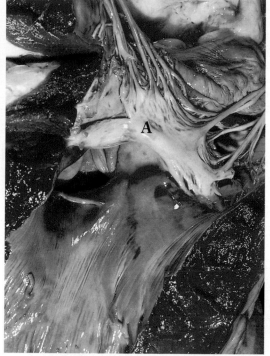

This two-day-old Friesian calf had a VSD (**23**). It was lethargic and dyspnoeic, especially on exercise, and had pronounced tachycardia, and showed hyperaemia of the muzzle. It died two days later.

In a severe case revealed at postmortem, note the patency of the ventricular septum (**24**). The position of the left atrioventricular (AV) valves (A) shows that the opening involves the fibrous portion of the septum. Small defects may produce few clinical effects except a loud systolic murmur. VSD may be combined with other cardiovascular anomalies.

Patent ductus arteriosus (PDA)

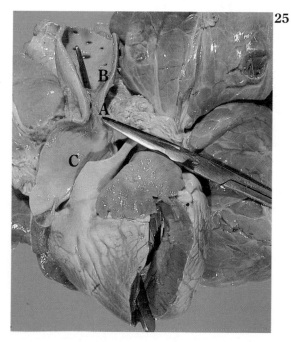

The heart of a crossbred Charolais bull calf (**25**), which suddenly collapsed with signs of severe tachypnoea when 18 days old, shows an opening (A) (internal diameter 2.5 mm) between the aortic trunk (B) and the pulmonary artery (C). This opening usually closes soon after birth. If it remains patent, unoxygenated blood can pass from the pulmonary trunk into the aorta, producing signs similar to a VSD. Scissors point to the PDA. Forceps have been placed between the left ventricle (bottom) and the aorta to show normal blood flow.

Erythropoietic porphyria ('pink tooth')

The teeth (**26**) and ribs (**27**) are brownish-red owing to an abnormal accumulation of uroporphyrin I. Porphyria results from a deficiency of the enzyme uroporphyrinogen III cosynthetase. The major signs, which include retarded growth, discolouration of the teeth and urine, pale mucosae, and photodermatitis, vary considerably with the age of the cattle and the season.

Diagnosis is aided by demonstration of ultraviolet (UV) fluorescence of the teeth. Affected cattle, if their retention can be justified economically for fattening, should be permanently housed. This rare condition is inherited as a simple autosomal recessive gene. *Differential diagnosis:* photosensitisation due to other causes (see pp. 30, 214, 215).

26

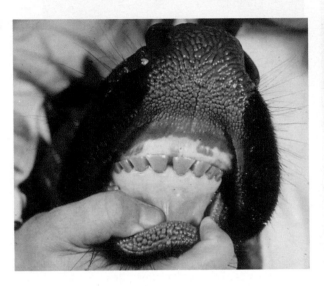

27

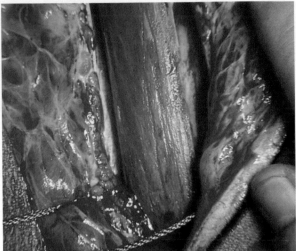

2 Neonatal disorders

Introduction

This chapter covers disorders of the calf from birth until postweaning. The first section deals with navel ill, umbilical hernia and general conditions of the navel. Later sections cover different forms of diarrhoea and alopecia, with a miscellaneous group including calf diphtheria and joint ill. According to the presenting signs, other diseases of the young calf are considered in the relevant chapters, for example, lice, ringworm and skin diseases are to be found in Chapter 3, respiratory problems in Chapter 5, and meningitis in Chapter 9.

A calf mortality rate of 5% of live births is considered to be a 'normal' figure. Much higher losses may occur where husbandry and management are poor. There are many reasons why the young calf is particularly susceptible to disease: its defence mechanisms are not fully developed; it will be going through the transition from passive to active immunity; it may have several changes of diet; and, moreover, the navel provides an additional route by which infection may enter the body. Many calf diseases are exacerbated by failure to provide adequate housing, management or colostral intake.

Conditions of the navel

Umbilical eventration

Umbilical eventration is seen in a small proportion of calves immediately after birth. The prolapsed intestines (jejunum) may be fully exposed, as in the Friesian (**28**), or contained in a sac of peritoneum. Opening the sac in a Charolais calf revealed a congested intestine (**29**). Often the exposed intestine ruptures when the calf moves. The prognosis is then hopeless. In more advanced and exposed cases the intestinal loops turn a deep red colour owing to ischaemic necrosis.

28
29

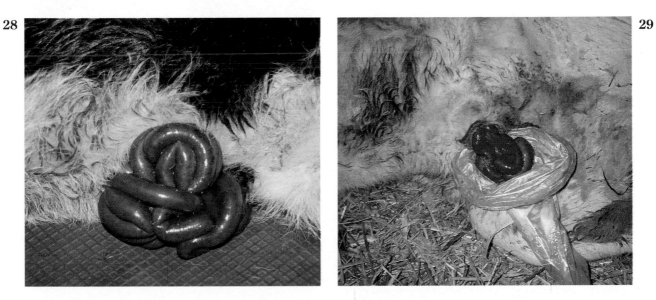

Navel ill (omphalophlebitis)

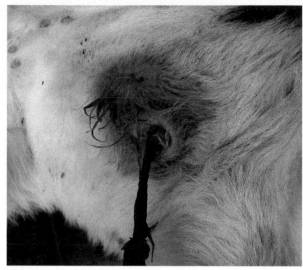

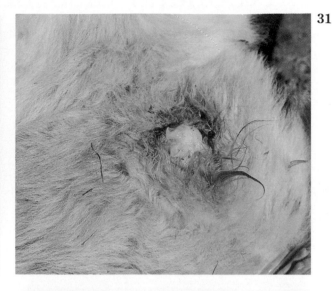

Lacking skin or any other protective layer, the moist, fleshy navel cord is particularly prone to infection until it dries up, normally within one week of birth. In the first calf (**30**) (shown at three days old) the enlarged, still moist navel cord is seen entering an inflamed and swollen umbilical ring. Navel ill is uncommon at this age.

The more typical case is pyrexic, with a swollen, painful navel exuding creamy-white pus (**31**). Culture usually reveals a mixed bacterial flora including *Escherichia coli*, *Proteus*, *Staphylococcus* and *Actinomyces pyogenes*. This case persisted for several weeks.

Alopecia on the medial aspects of the thighs (**32**) is due to a combination of urine scald and excessive cleansing of the navel by the owner. Some cases show no gross discharge, but the tip of the swollen navel will be moist, having a purulent smell. Septicaemia can result in localisation of infection in the joints (**65 & 66**), meninges, endocardium or end-arteries of limbs. *Differential diagnosis:* this includes umbilical hernia (**34**), eventration (**28**) and granuloma (**33**).

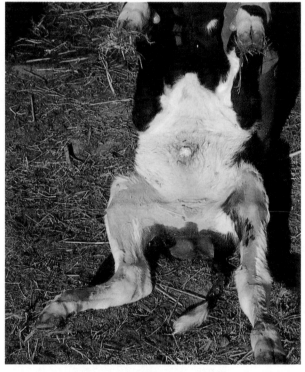

Umbilical granuloma

A small, nonpurulent mass of granulation tissue protrudes from the navel of this two-week-old crossbred Hereford (**33**). It is only slightly painful and the calf is not pyrexic, but the condition will not resolve until the mass is removed by ligation at its base.

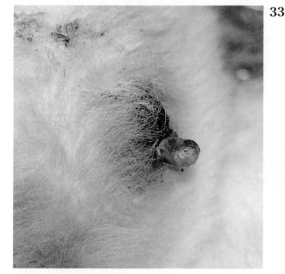

Umbilical hernia

A large, soft, painless and fluctuating swelling can be seen cranial to the prepuce in this three-month-old Friesian male calf (**34**). Hair has been clipped from the skin overlying the hernial sac, within which the small intestine and the fibrosed navel cord were palpable. Both were easily reducible through the large umbilical ring. Although present from birth, many hernias are not noticed until the calf is at least 2–3 weeks old. A proportion of cases are inherited. *Differential diagnosis:* navel abscess (**35**), urolithiasis and ruptured urethra (see **498**).

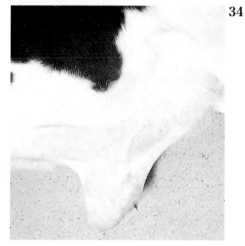

Umbilical abscess

The swelling in this four-month-old Friesian male (**35**) is cranial to the prepuce (compare urolithiasis (**498**), where it is caudal) and appeared spontaneously. The mass was initially hard, hot and painful. Pyrexia led to systemic illness. Parenteral antibiotics resulted in a change to a more fluctuating swelling, which was successfully lanced and drained.

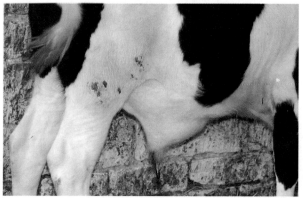

A hernia and an umbilical abscess can occur together. Occasionally, navel ill or navel abscess produces a localised peritonitis that erodes through the rumen wall to produce a rumenal fistula. Sometimes, large abscesses develop intra-abdominally along the course of an infected umbilical vein (omphalophleb-itis) and spread to the liver. **36** shows a three-month-old Friesian male with a grossly enlarged navel sac, soiled anteriorly. Rumen contents leaked through the fistula, shown in close-up in **37**. *Differential diagnosis:* navel ill (**30**), umbilical hernia (**34**) and rectourethral fistula (**38**).

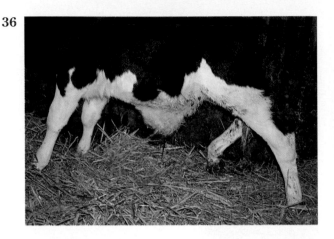

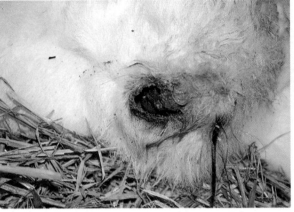

Rectourethral fistula

Note the very soiled hair around the navel and prepuce, and the discoloured urine in this two-day-old Holstein male (**38**). This uncommon condition may be confused with navel ill and pervious urachus.

Navel suckling

Navel suckling (**39**) is a common vice in group-housed, bucket-fed calves. The calf being sucked has an enlarged navel which could be infected, and there is hair loss around the navel, indicating a chronic problem. The ears, tail and scrotum are also suckled.

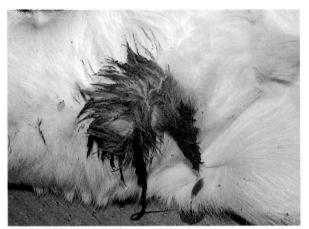

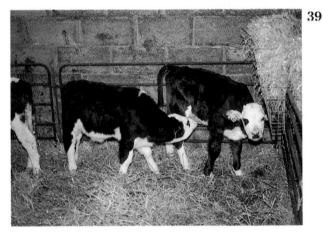

Calf Scour

Enteritis and diarrhoea in calves are major causes of death in the first few weeks of life. A wide range of agents can be involved, some producing diarrhoea with or without dehydration, others leading to systemic involvement. Diarrhoea in the first few days of life is commonly caused by bacterial infections, for example, *E. coli* or *Clostridium welchii*. Their toxins lead to hypersecretion from the intestine and subsequent fluid loss, seen as diarrhoea. Viral infections (rotavirus and coronavirus) and *Cryptosporidia* typically occur at 10–14 days (as maternal colostral antibody wanes) and are considered to be the major causes of calf scour. Diarrhoea occurs because the intestinal wall is damaged, preventing reabsorption of fluid. *Salmonella* scouring can occur at any age. Vaccines are available against *E. coli*, rotavirus and *Salmonella*. Hygiene and good feeding practices are very important for control. It is not possible to differentiate fully between the various causes of scour on the basis of gross appearance alone, although the following illustrations give a few guidelines.

Rotavirus and cryptosporidia

40

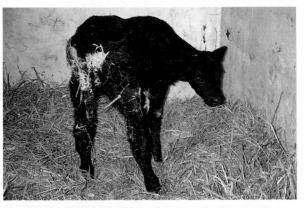

41

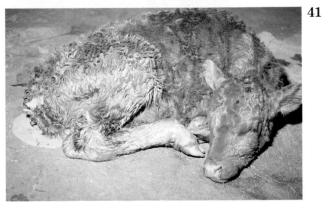

42

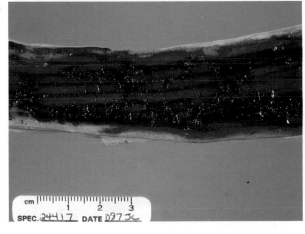

The majority of calves become infected with rotavirus, coronavirus and *Cryptosporidia*, but normally only those subjected to a heavy challenge or concurrent disease show clinical signs. The Limousin calf (**40**) is bright and alert, but has a pasty yellow diarrhoea around the tail. Both rotavirus and *Cryptosporidia* were identified in the faeces. More advanced cases (**41**) show dehydration and general systemic involvement such as sunken eyes, a dry muzzle, hyperaemia of the nares and a purulent nasal discharge. At postmortem two days later, the colon was thickened, corrugated and exuding blood (**42**). *Cryptosporidia*, rotavirus, coronavirus and enterotoxigenic *E. coli* (responsible for the haemorrhagic colitis) were all isolated.

White scour

White scour occurs when intestinal damage is such that partially digested white milk is passed in the faeces. Note the characteristic white faecal soiling of the flanks and tail in this two-week-old Holstein heifer (**43**). Originally considered to be part of the colibacillosis syndrome, it is now known that white scour can result from a range of agents, including rotavirus. **44** shows the voluminous, white, rotavirus-positive faeces voided during an explosive outbreak in a calf unit.

43

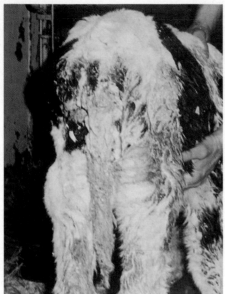

44

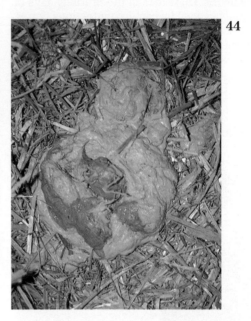

Enterotoxaemia

Clostridium welchii enterotoxaemia normally affects calves in the first few days of life. The small intestine on the left of **45** shows a dark-red ischaemic necrosis. Other areas are gas-filled, which is indicative of gut stasis and gas formation. Following sudden death, type C enterotoxin was demonstrated.

45

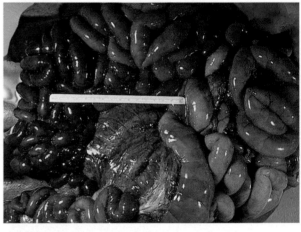

Salmonellosis

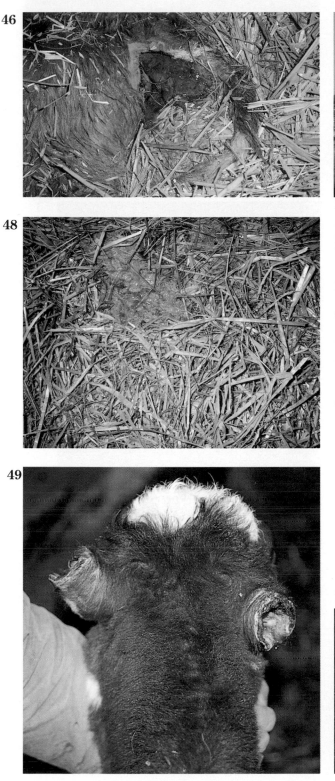

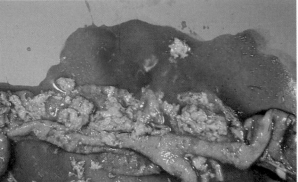

46 shows a week-old crossbred Hereford calf that is moribund and passing dysenteric faeces, a mixture of blood, mucus and intestinal mucosal lining. Classically, a postmortem revealed a diphtheritic enteritis (**47**), with thickening of the mucosa. However, not all calves are affected so severely. Although *Salmonella typhimurium* was isolated from the dysenteric faeces in **48**, the affected calf, a three-week-old Friesian, was only mildly ill. Other cases show slight intestinal inflammation, the main changes being lung congestion and epicardial and renal haemorrhages. Animals recovering from peracute septicaemia (especially *S. dublin*) may occasionally develop necrosis of the extremities, particularly in the ear tips and legs. The four-month-old Friesian (**49**) was recovering from a nonspecific pyrexia six weeks previously. Ear-tip necrosis has produced a bilateral slough of more than half of the pinna. *S. dublin* was isolated from the faeces. In the four-month-old crossbred Hereford (**50**), circumferential skin necrosis immediately above the hind fetlocks has produced gangrene and necrosis of the extremities. There may be over-extension at the fetlocks, probably due to flexor tendon rupture. Salivation is a pain response. *Differential diagnosis: E. coli* septicaemia (p.21), coccidiosis (**55**) and ergot poisoning (**402**).

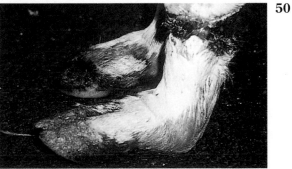

Abomasal ulceration

Bucket-fed calves commonly develop ulcers, possibly associated with irregular feeding and early consumption of dry food. The majority pass unrecognised. The two-week-old Friesian in **51** was moribund, with drooping ears, sunken eyes and regurgitated rumen contents on its lips. It died within hours and a post-mortem revealed an acute abomasitis with two perforated ulcers (**52**), each with a creamy-white necrotic lining. Death was due to acute peritonitis (**53**). Fibrin and food coat the serosal surface of an inflamed and dilated small intestine. Abomasal ulcers are also seen in adult cattle (**192–194**).

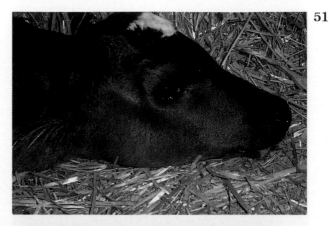

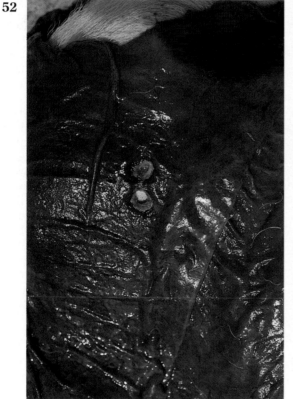

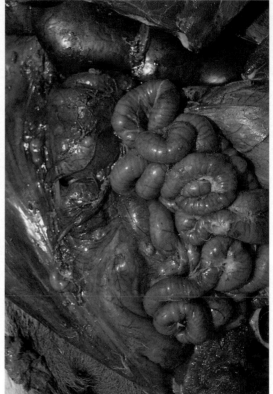

Coccidiosis

Coccidiosis is an infection of the lower small intestine, caecum, colon and rectum, caused by the protozoan parasite *Eimeria zuernii* or *E. bovis*. It is usually associated with calves crowded in unhygienic conditions. Adult animals (e.g., suckler cows) may be carriers. Affected calves are dull, pyrexic and typically produce

54

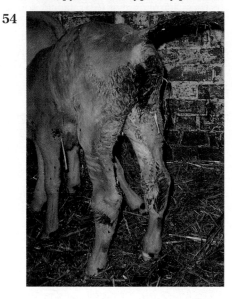

watery faeces, usually mixed with blood. Tenesmus (**54**), with continued straining and passing of small quantities of blood and faeces, is a characteristic sign. The anal sphincter is open, exposing the rectal mucosa. Hair loss on the inside of the leg results from faecal soiling. **55** shows a thickened and inflamed colonic mucosa from another case. Blood on the surface of freshly passed faeces is a normal feature of some calves, but it occurs more often following stress, e.g., transport, or sale through a livestock market. *Differential diagnosis*: includes salmonellosis (**46**).

55

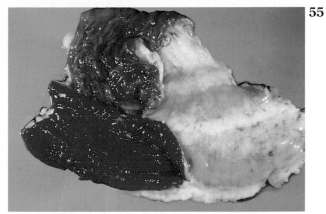

Ruminal tympany and digestive scour

Chronic ruminal tympany and scour that occur immediately pre- and postweaning, commonly result from feeding errors that produce incomplete oesophageal groove closure. Milk entering the rumen may produce bloat with severe colic. Inadequate intakes of concentrates preweaning may also retard ruminal development. The four-week-old Charolais calf (**56**) shows faecal soiling of the tail and perineum, associated with

56

chronic diarrhoea which often accompanies the condition. The bloated rumen has blood at the site of an attempted trocarisation. Bloat also occurs in older cattle (see **180**). The seven-week-old white Friesian calf in the centre of **57** is in poor condition, with its tail and perineum matted with faeces due to chronic digestive scour. These calves were fed unsuitable protein in a concentrate intended for adult cattle and remained stunted for many months. Infection with *Campylobacter* species has been implicated in other cases.

57

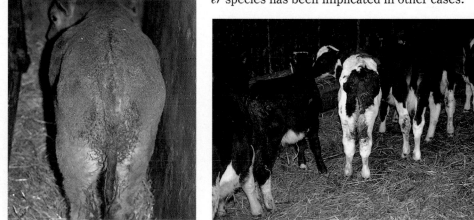

Alopecia

Three distinct types of alopecia in calves are illustrated.

Idiopathic alopecia

Spontaneous hair loss often occurs over the head, as in the crossbred Hereford calf (**58**). Less commonly, the whole body may be involved. Milk allergy and vitamin E deficiency are suggested causes. Most cases recover slowly over 1–2 months, without treatment.

Alopecia post-diarrhoea

In the Charolais calf (**59**), faecal soiling following severe rotavirus scour has totally denuded the perineum and ventral surface of the tail. Following recumbency, there may also be further hair loss over the hock and lower abdomen, including the navel. Urine scald may also be a contributory cause (**32**).

58

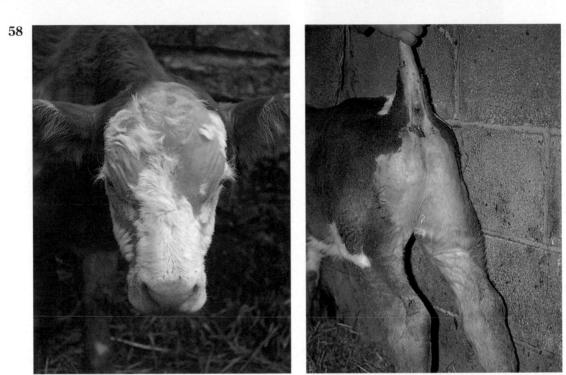

59

Alopecia on the muzzle

Alopecia of this type is seen in calves fed milk substitute and results from fat globules adhering to the skin over the muzzle. The causes include inadequate mixing of milk substitute, feeding it at too low a temperature, and calves that drink slowly. Hair loss on this three-week-old crossbred Hereford (**60**) extends from the muzzle onto the nasal arch. The underlying pink skin shows secondary scab formation.

60

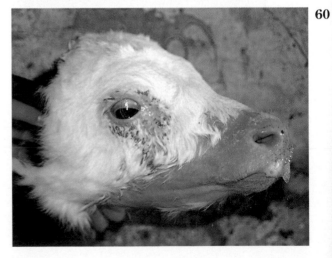

Miscellaneous disorders

Diphtheria (oral necrobacillosis)

This ulcerative necrosis of the cheek, tongue, pharynx or larynx is caused by *Fusobacterium necrophorum* and can produce a range of clinical signs. The Charolais calf (**61**) is a mild case involving the cheek and producing an external swelling and oral mucosal ulceration. If the tongue is involved, calves salivate excessively (**62**). They may drool and regurgitate partially masticated food. **63** shows a deep ulcerative area on the tongue that has been cleaned to remove necrotic debris and food. A few calves develop laryngeal diphtheria, manifested as a severe dyspnoea, stridor ('roaring' breathing) and pyrexia. Such calves otherwise remain surprisingly bright and continue to feed, thus differentiating the condition from pneumonia. Normally, there is no palpable external laryngeal swelling. Postmortem examination (**64**) reveals a caseous infection (A), typically located bilaterally between the vocal processes (B) and the medial angles of the arytenoid cartilages (C), where it restricts air passage.

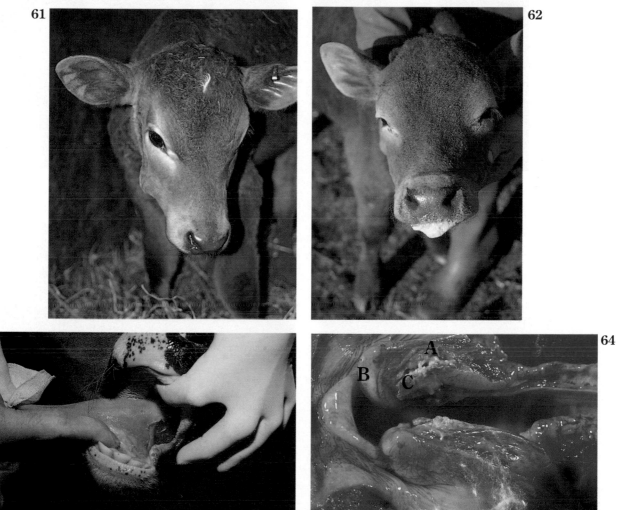

Joint ill

Septicaemic infection entering the navel at birth may localise in joints to produce arthritis and severe lameness, especially in colostrum-deficient calves. In the Friesian calf (65) the carpus is swollen as a result of intra-articular fibrinopurulent material and a periarticular soft-tissue reaction. These changes are seen in the opened hock joints in 66. The articular cartilage had remained undamaged. Affected calves are pyrexic. The hock, carpus and stifle are most commonly involved. Polyarthritis is often fatal. Joint ill is first seen at 3–4 weeks old (later than navel ill) and typical cases have no residual evidence of navel infection. *Differential diagnosis*: physeal separation (367).

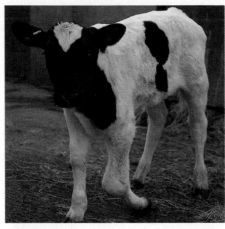

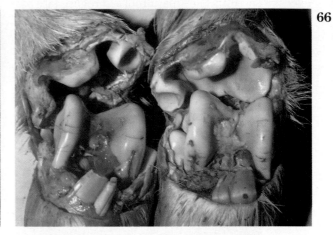

Iodine deficiency goitre

Pregnant cows have an increased iodine requirement and deficient animals may give birth to stillborn or weakly calves with enlarged thyroids (> 20g), known as goitre. A subcutaneous swelling is clearly visible over the larynx in this two-week-old Zebu calf from Brazil (67), but in the vast majority of cases there are no external signs and the thyroid glands must be dissected and weighed. Oedema and hair loss may also occur. Iodine-deficient soils occur in granite areas, mountainous regions and areas distant from the sea.

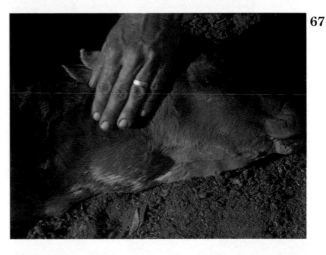

3 Integumentary disorders

Introduction

Skin is the largest organ of the body and performs a wide range of functions. It is mechanically protective against physical injury and provides a barrier against infections, many of which only become established when surface integrity has been compromised by physical or environmental trauma. Sense receptors detect touch and pain. Vitamin D is synthesised under the influence of ultraviolet light. Skin has a primary function in heat control, insulating against heat and cold, and, through sweating, it acts as a thermoregulator. The depth and thickness of hair coat is the main factor affecting insulation.

The major breeds of cattle in Europe and North America are derived from *Bos taurus* and have a limited ability to sweat. Cattle derived from *Bos indicus* (Brahman, USA; Africander, Africa), such as the Santa Gertrudis, can sweat copiously for long periods, although there are considerable differences in sweat production from different regions of the body surface.

Visual appraisal of the skin is easily carried out and a wide range of disorders is recognised. Anaphylactic reactions can produce urticaria. Photosensitisation may result from a range of intoxications including St. John's Wort, *Lantana* and facial eczema (see also Chapter 13, **710, 719–721**). Parasitic infections (lice and mange), fungal infections (ringworm), fly infestations (myiasis and warbles) and bacterial infections (skin tuberculosis) all produce skin changes which are discussed in this chapter. The final section deals with physical conditions such as haematomas, abscesses, frostbite and other traumatic incidents. Many skin changes are secondary to other diseases and these are described in the relevant chapters, for example, gangrene secondary to mastitis (see **587**) or ergot poisoning (see **402**), or subcutaneous swellings associated with urolithiasis (see **498**) or umbilical (navel) conditions (**34**).

Cutaneous urticaria (urticaria, angioneurotic oedema, 'blaine')

Thought to be a plant or immunological hypersensitivity reaction, urticaria is sudden in onset. The Friesian cow (**68**) has raised plaques of oedema (wheals) over the face and shoulders. The eyelids and muzzle are swollen. Although looking depressed, she was eating well and, like many such mild cases, recovered within 36 hours. The Simmental cow (**69**) was a much more advanced case. She was pyrexic and in considerable pain. The head, grossly enlarged due to subcutaneous oedema, was often rested on the ground. The skin of the muzzle is hyperaemic. Localised areas sloughed a few weeks later. Some cases are due to snake bites or bee stings.

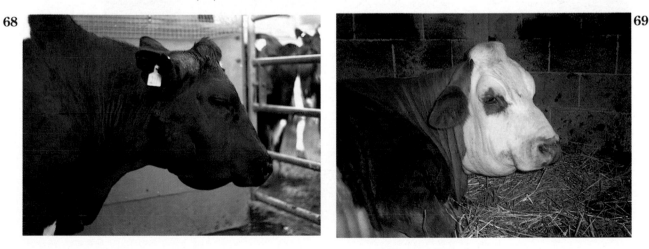

68   69

Photosensitisation (photosensitive dermatitis)

70

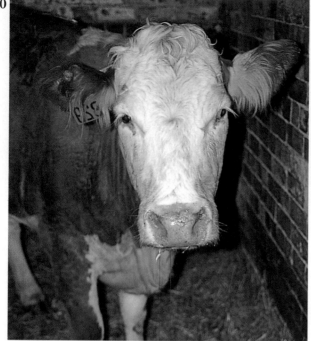

Photosensitisation has a worldwide occurrence. Photoreactive agents accumulating under the skin convert ultraviolet light into thermal energy, leading to inflammatory changes that initially produce skin swelling and, later, a possible slough. Only white or lightly pigmented skin is affected, since black skin prevents absorption of sunlight. The initial photoreactive agent may have been ingested (primary photosensitisation), or may be produced as a result of liver damage (hepatogenous). In cattle the principle agents are porphyrins and phylloerythrins, the latter being a normal breakdown product of chlorophyll that is not metabolised further. Liver damage may result from ingestion of a wide range of drugs, plants or chemicals.

In the early stages, affected animals show discomfort and pyrexia, with erythema and encrustation around the margins of the nostrils (**70**) and erythema of the teats (**71**), as in this Simmental cow. The teats are very painful and may later blister and slough (**72**), making milking almost impossible. The thickness of the skin slough, in this case only moderate, depends on the degree of initial damage. The primary febrile

71

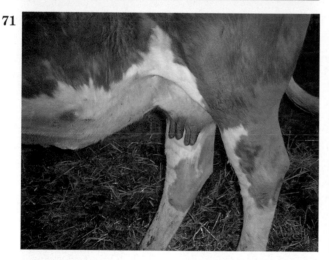

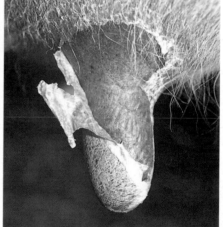

72

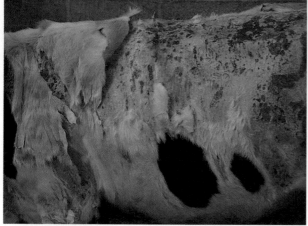

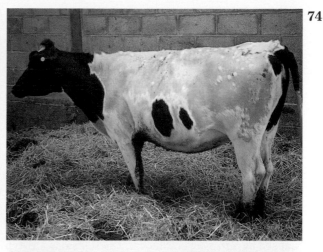

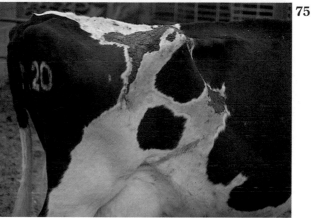

phase, oedema and thickening of the white skin had passed unnoticed in the heifer in **73**, and she was presented with sloughing of dry, hard areas of white skin and with a new epidermis forming beneath. Seven weeks later (**74**) the new skin was well-developed. Hair regrowth was possible owing to the preservation of hair follicles deeper in the epidermis. Areas of granulation tissue may retard healing (**75**), especially over bony prominences such as the pelvis. A dry dermatitis persisted in this cow for a further two years. The condition also occurs in *Lantana* poisoning (**710**) and facial eczema (**719–721**). *Differential diagnosis:* foot- and-mouth-disease (**629–633**), bluetongue (**641**), bovine herpes mammillitis (**597**) and vesicular stomatitis (**604**).

Brown coat colour

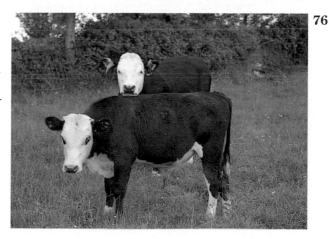

Copper deficiency affects several systems (see **410–414**), but classically causes loss of coat colour. However, copper deficiency is not the only cause of brown coat colour. Animals turned out to spring grazing may retain their winter coat (**76**), particularly younger calves and first-lactation heifers. Although grazing the same pasture, the older animal at the rear is not affected. *Differential diagnosis*: molybdenum toxicosis (**730**).

Parasitic skin conditions

Cattle are affected by four genera of mange mites, i.e., *Sarcoptes, Chorioptes, Psoroptes* and *Demodex*, six species of lice, skin helminths (*Stephanofilaria* and *Parafilaria*), myiasis (screw-worm) and various fly infestations. Many such conditions cannot be differentiated on clinical examination alone and laboratory tests are necessary. Often, several conditions coexist, e.g., mange, ringworm and lice may occur simultaneously on cattle in poor condition. The appearance and location of mange lesions are generally characteristic for the particular mite, although specific diagnosis depends on microscopic examination of the mouthparts.

Mange

Sarcoptic mange (scabies)

Caused by *Sarcoptes scabiei* var. *bovis*, lesions are typically seen over the head, neck and hindquarters (**77**). Note the hair loss and severe thickening of the skin in **78**. The white areas show secondary damage due to rubbing. In severe cases there may be almost total hair loss. The close-up view (**79**) shows the dry, scaly appearance of the thickened skin.

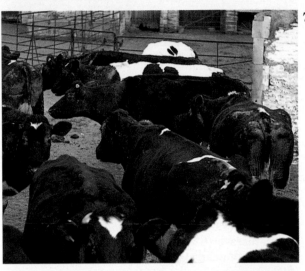

77

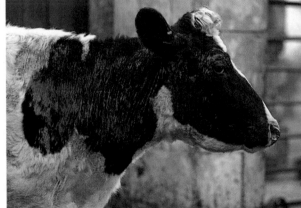

78

79

Chorioptic mange

Chorioptic mange is the most common type of mange in cattle. The fold of skin beside the tail is the characteristic site for infestation by *Chorioptes bovis* (**80**). Lesions comprise a thick encrustation overlying an area of moist, serous exudate. They are intensely irritant. In more advanced cases (**81**) red, pustular lesions may spread down the perineum.

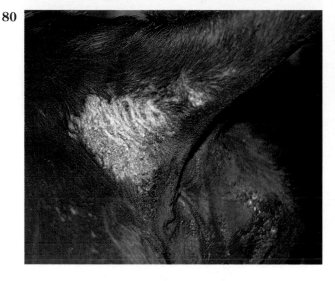

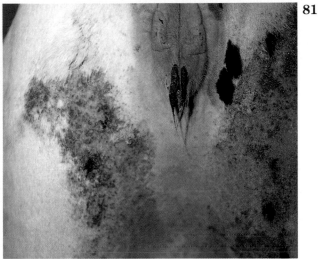

Psoroptic mange

Note the skin thickening and hair loss in the Guernsey cow (**82**), extending from the vulva to the udder. The condition may start at the withers and spread over the whole body. Pruritus may be marked. Psoroptic mange is notifiable in North America, where eradication programmes have been in progress for many years. One type of mite that causes this sort of mange is *Psoroptes nululensis*. Another, *Psoroptes ovis*, also attacks sheep and horses.

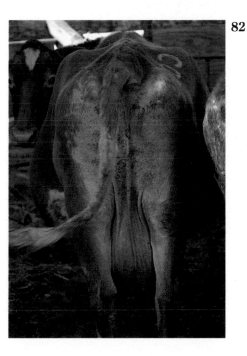

Demodectic mange (follicular mange)

Small papules are seen on the white skin of this cow (**83**), from which a thick, white, waxy material containing large numbers of mites can be expressed. Some nodules become secondarily infected with *Staphylococci*. The condition is generally mild, with a spontaneous recovery. Extensive hair loss is rare.

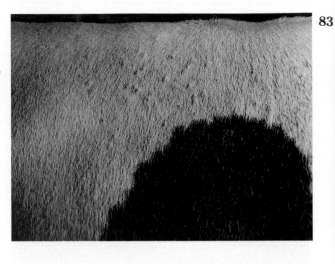

Lice (pediculosis)

Sucking lice (for example, *Haematopinus eurysternus* and *Linognathus vituli* and, in North America, *Solenopotes capillatus*) are slower-moving than biting lice (*Bovicola bovis*). In addition to pruritus (the only lesion due to biting lice), they may produce severe anaemia, loss of condition and even death. Parting the white hair along the withers (**84**) reveals small, brown lice, just visible to the naked eye. Lice are often also seen on the scrotum.

Clinically, infestations are manifested by rubbing, biting or scratching. In **85** the calf's tongue is protruding and its head is held on one side, a stance typical of pruritus. In early cases the hair develops vertical lines, and small, hairless areas with white scurf may arise from biting. In more advanced cases (**85 & 86**) the skin is thickened round the eyes and muzzle and the vertical hair lines on the neck are thrown into

84

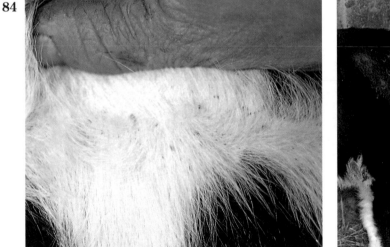

85

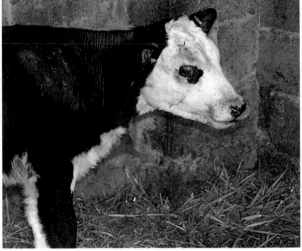

thick folds (**86**). The calf in **86** was also stunted and anaemic. Ringworm often occurs in association with lice. Early lesions are seen on the shoulder in **85**. Pale beige-coloured oval lice eggs, glued onto the hair shafts, can often be seen with the naked eye, particularly on the tip of the ear (**87**). In older animals the coat may be matted with lice eggs. Eggs hatch over a period of 2–3 weeks.

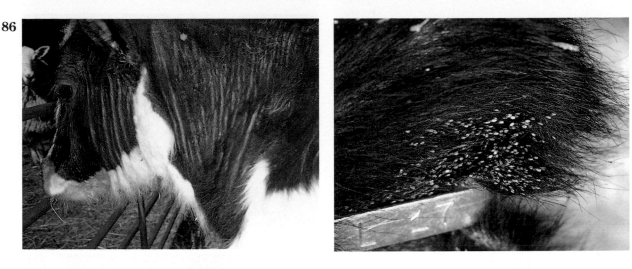

Ringworm (dermatophytosis)

Ringworm is a fungal infection of the superficial, dead, keratinised tissues of the hair and skin, of which *Trichophyton verrucosum* is the most common cause in cattle. Occasionally, *Microsporum* species may be involved. Lesions are commonly seen over the head and neck (**88**), but they may occur on any part of the body. They consist of circular areas of alopecia in which the skin is thickened and often markedly encrusted. The initial stages show progressive alopecia and erythema of the skin, with encrustation developing later. Lesions expand from the periphery and several smaller areas may coalesce (**89**).

Ringworm causes irritation and if affected calves rub against posts or feed troughs, they deposit spores that can remain infective for up to four years.

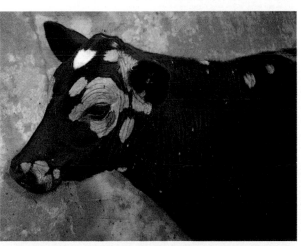

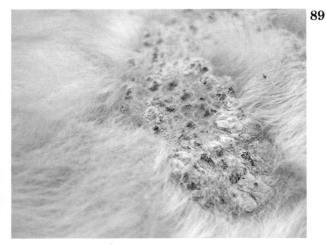

Skin helminths

Cattle are affected by four genera of skin helminths, *Onchocerca*, *Pelodera* (*Rhabditis bovis*), *Stephanofilaria* and *Parafilaria*.

Cutaneous stephanofilariasis

Microfilariae of *Stephanofilaria stilesi* are introduced into the skin of the ventral midline by the horn fly (*Haematobia irritans*) as it feeds, producing large, circular areas of dermatitis, seen here on the ventral abdomen (**90**). Recent lesions are moist, with blood or serous exudate, whilst long-standing areas are characterised by alopecia and hyperkeratosis.

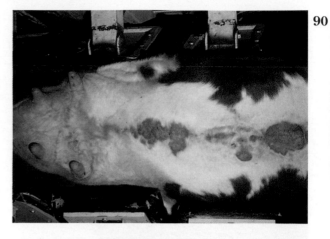
90

Stephanofilarial otitis (parasitic otitis)

Caused by *Stephanofilaria zaheeri*, parasitic otitis is most prevalent in older cattle in humid weather. Note the painful erythematous inflammation on the inside of the ear of this Zebu cow from India (**91**). In East Africa a free-living nematode, *Rhabditis bovis*, can also produce a purulent otitis that may lead to middle ear involvement.

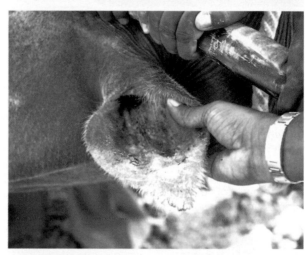
91

Stephanofilarial dermatitis (hump sore)

Transmitted by flies, *Stephanofilaria assamensis* produces an irritant dermatitis. The raw, granulating areas seen on the hump of this Zebu cow from India (**92**) result in lost milk production, reduced working capacity and hide damage. Exotic cattle are affected more than indigenous breeds.

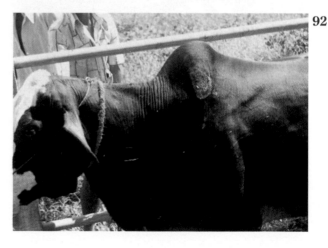
92

Parafilarial infection

Transmitted by flies of the *Musca* genus, *Parafilaria bovicola* produces painful subcutaneous lesions that may impede the productivity of draught animals, but, more importantly, can lead to serious economic losses from carcase trimming of beef cattle at slaughter. The female worm perforates the host's skin and oviposits into blood dripping from the wound. A typical 'bleeding spot' is illustrated on the chest of this South Afri-can bull (**93**). (The faecal soiling on the crest of the neck is coincidental.) Flies feeding on the blood, which may continue to flow for several hours, ingest eggs containing microfilariae. A typical female worm nodule is shown in **94**, closely adherent to the hide.

Parafilarial infection is common in parts of Asia, Africa and Europe, and fly control, including impregnated ear tags, is important in prevention.

93
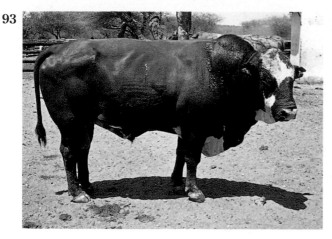

94
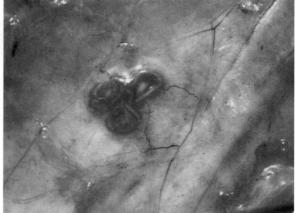

Besnoitiosis

A sporozoan parasite of the family Sarcocystidae, *Besnoitia besnoiti* can cause a systemic illness of fever, diarrhoea and lymphadenopathy, or, as in this case (**95**), a dry dermatitis. The South African bull shows intense thickening of the skin and complete hair loss over the affected areas. In advanced cases the skin may crack, predisposing the animal to secondary bacterial infection or myiasis, and a resulting weight loss. Besnoitiosis has been reported in Southern Europe, Africa, Asia and South America.

95
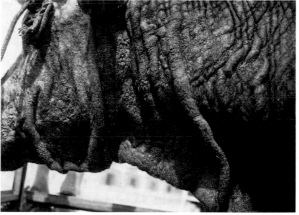

Dermatophilosis (cutaneous papillomatosis, streptothricosis)

In temperate climates, where lesions are mild, infection with the bacterium *Dermatophilus congolensis* develops following exposure to prolonged periods of wet weather. The lesions in the Friesian cow (**96**) are nonpruritic, raised clumps of hair (which can be easily lifted off) with a light brown, waxy exudate at the bsse. In warmer climates, particularly during periods of high humidity and increased fly and tick activity, zoospores dormant in the epidermis may become active in almost epidemic proportions to cause more severe skin damage, with secondary inflammation. These cattle from Antigua (**97 & 98**) show small, raised, nodular skin tufts, especially over the neck and shoulders. More advanced lesions coalesce to form plaques (**99**) with an almost wart-like appearance. *Differential diagnosis*: warble fly (**104 & 105**) and lumpy-skin disease (**648**).

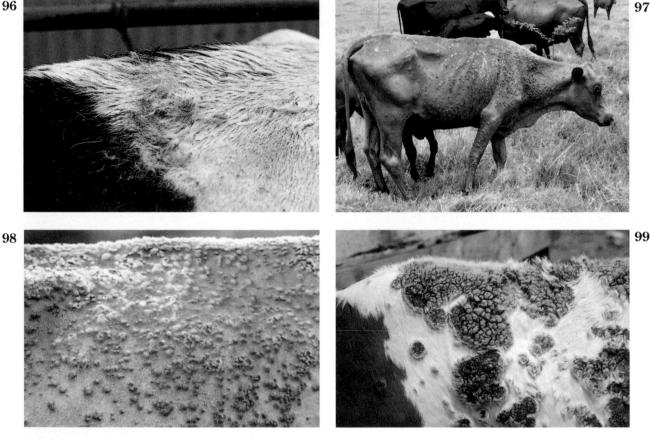

96

97

98

99

Fibropapillomatosis (papillomatosis, warts)

Warts, predominantly seen in 6–18-month-old cattle, appear as fleshy lumps on the head and neck. Large, pendulous warts may also be seen along the brisket and sternum. Their size varies enormously, from 5 cm in diameter (**100**) to small nodules, only just visible above the hair of the skin. Warts also occur on teats (**605–607**), the penis (**510**), and in the bladder (**701**), when they are associated with bracken poisoning. Skin warts are caused by papovaviruses. Five species have been reported, including three distinct species on teats. Flies and lice may be important in transmission. Typically, warts resolve spontaneously following development of viral immunity.

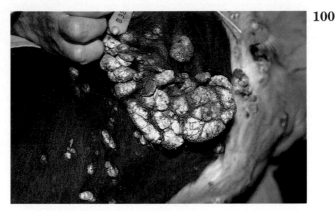

100

Skin tuberculosis (atypical mycotuberculosis)

Typical indurated nodules, running along the path of corded lymphatics beneath the skin, are visible on the lateral aspect of the foreleg and the shoulder (**101**). The lesions contain nonpathogenic, acid-fast bacteria. Affected animals may react positively to the tuberculin test. *Differential diagnosis*: ulcerative lymphangitis (**102**) and bovine farcy.

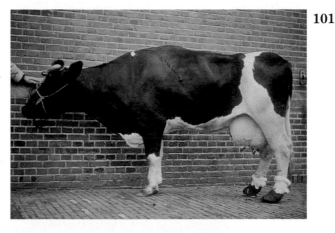

101

Ulcerative lymphangitis (pseudotuberculosis)

Caused by *Actinomyces* (*Corynebacterium*) *pseudotuberculosis*, ulcerative lymphangitis is primarily a condition of sheep and goats, although cattle can be affected. Large, caseous nodules occur in the lymphatics of the lower limb (**102**) and may involve drainage lymph nodes.

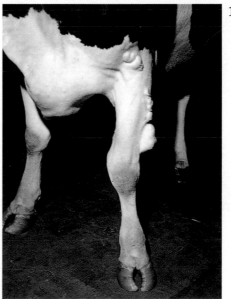

102

Fly infestations

A wide range of fly species feeds on cattle, the most common being horn flies, buffalo flies (*Haematobia irritans*) (seen on the skin of the back in **103**), head flies (*Hydrotea irritans*) and face flies (*Musca autumnalis*). In addition to causing annoyance, and therefore restricting feed intake, these flies may also produce anaemia and transmit disease, for example, *Parafilaria* and *Moraxella bovis* in infectious bovine keratoconjunctivitis (IBK).

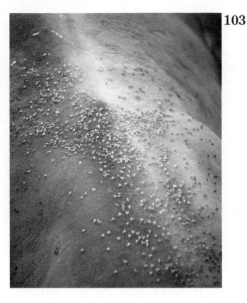

103

Warble fly

There are two species of warble fly: *Hypoderma bovis* and *H. lineatum*. Both lay eggs on the hair of the lower legs. Emerging larvae penetrate the dermis and migrate to the skin of the back, which they puncture for breathing holes, and then encyst. Encysted larvae produce smooth skin swellings (**104**) known as warbles. Over a period of 4–6 weeks, warble larvae undergo three moults, changing from white to black, the third-stage larva then emerging through the breathing hole to fall to the ground to pupate. In (**105**) a late third stage larva has been manually expressed onto the skin, over the anterior chest. A cluster of five larval breathing holes, with larvae feeding beneath, is present in the skin, dorsal to the lumbar spine. Losses due to warbles arise from damage to the most valuable part of the hide, from reduced grazing due to fear of the adult fly, and rare cases of paralysis resulting from hypersensitivity to dead larvae in the spinal canal. Warbles is a notifiable disease in Britain.

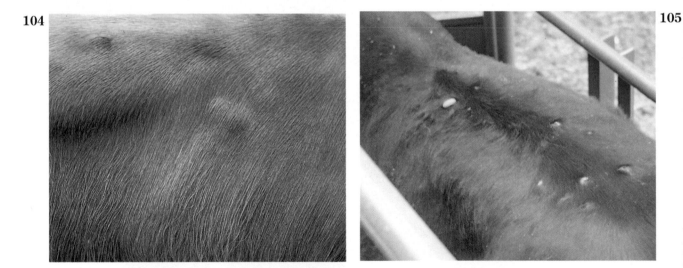

104

105

Tropical warble fly: *Dermatobia hominis*

Dermatobia hominis is known as the tropical warble fly. It is found only in Southern Mexico and Central and South America, where it is a major problem. Human infection can also occur. The adult lays its eggs on a range of other insects (49 different species have been recorded), which then transmit the eggs to cattle when feeding on them. Eggs are visible between the wings of the fly, *Musca domestica*, in **106**. On hatching, larvae burrow through the skin and encyst to form a subcutaneous nodule, the warble. Firm warble nodules are seen on the Hereford crossbred cow from Brazil (**107**), especially over the shoulders and flanks. (Warbles of *Hypoderma* are seen only along the back, **104**.) After feeding for 40–50 days, the mature larvae emerge (**108**) and fall to the ground to pupate. Severe pain and irritation, with secondary infection, may occur as the larvae emerge, as seen in the Zebu cow in **109**.

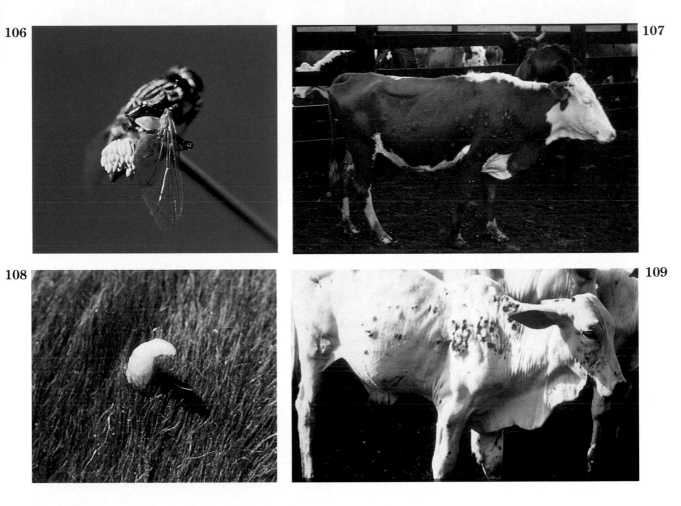

106 107 108 109

Screw-worm or myiasis

The parasites known as screw-worms are the larvae of the blowflies *Cochliomyia hominivorax* and *Chrysomya bezziana*. The adult fly lays eggs on wounds, the navel of neonates, or on tick-damaged areas (**653**, p.195). **110** shows an early infestation. More advanced lesions (**111**) may be filled with larvae of mixed ages, some of which will be mature and ready to leave and pupate in the soil. The disease is of major importance in South America and has been reported in North Africa.

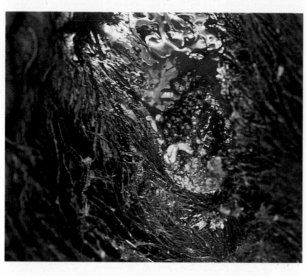

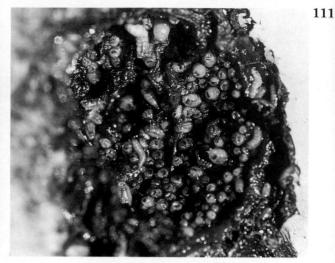

Traumatic and physical conditions

In addition to being the largest organ of the body, the skin is also the most exposed. Injury is common, particularly when cattle are housed in poorly designed, overcrowded buildings and handled roughly. Damp, dirty conditions may compromise the skin defences. When such factors are combined with inadequate bedding and projections from housing, abscesses or more severe injuries can result. Cattle can withstand wide extremes of temperature, although frostbite does occur. Haematomas are commonly the result of physical injury, whilst other subcutaneous swellings may result from hernia or rupture.

Haematoma

Haematomas are initially soft, painless, fluctuating, fluid-filled swellings that appear suddenly. Common sites are points where bruising of the skin against bone can occur, e.g., over the pelvic prominences (**112**) and spine (**113**), and on the flank (**114**) and

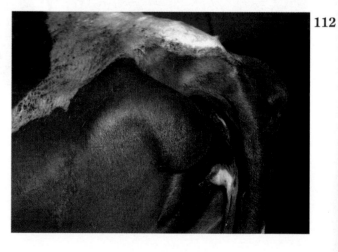

shoulder. The case in **113** occurred as a result of being trapped under a cubicle (free stall) division, and the flank haematoma (**114**) followed a horn gore. Without rupturing, the majority of smaller haematomas resolve to leave thick skin folds. Sometimes a haematoma becomes infected and develops into an abscess. Occasionally, haematomas burst, releasing the blood clot. In one such case, characteristic thick folds of skin can be seen cranial to the stifle (**115**).

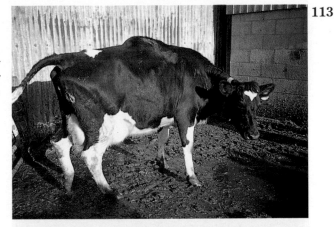

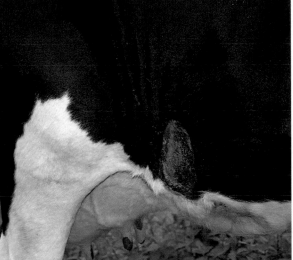

Bursitis of the neck

In **116**, hair loss at the cranial aspect of the lesion indicates that the bursitis was caused by continually pushing against a feed barrier. Like a haematoma, the swelling is soft, painless and fluctuating, but it develops more slowly. Aspiration disclosed a clear fluid.

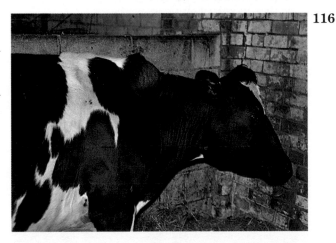

Skin abscesses

Abscesses are generally hard, hot, and slightly painful swellings that develop and enlarge slowly, thus differentiating them from a haematoma (**112**) or a hernia (**119**). The Hereford steer (**117**) has a sterile abscess on its neck, caused by the injection of a vaccine. Injecting a 40% solution of calcium borogluconate subcutaneously can lead to a hard, fluid-filled, sterile swelling developing over a period of 3–6 weeks. The popliteal region is a common site for abscessation, as seen in the Friesian cow (**118**). A large, fluctuating swelling is seen on the left leg, lateral to the stifle. The abscess is often deep in the muscle and may slowly enlarge over several months. Abscesses must be lanced and drained to achieve resolution.

117

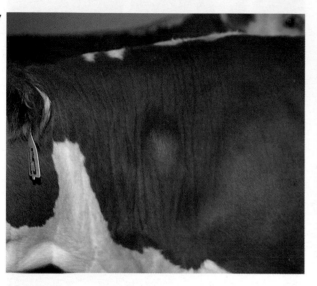

118

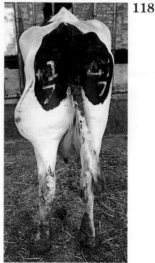

Flank hernia

The flank hernia in the Ayrshire cow (**119**) developed suddenly, probably as a result of a horn gore by another cow, two months before presentation. A second abdominal hernia is a more discrete swelling of the lower left flank in a yearling calf (**120**). The aetiology was again traumatic. The oblique scar is a result of the original perforating injury. The hernial contents were reducible. Surgery, including a mesh implant, was successful.

119

120

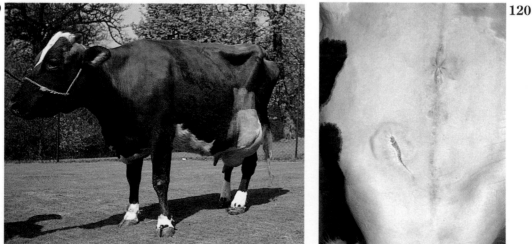

Rupture of prepubic tendon

The udder has dropped ventrally and the sac of skin and muscle anterior to it contains abdominal organs (**121**). Hydrallantois had resulted in the excessive abdominal distension and subsequent rupture.

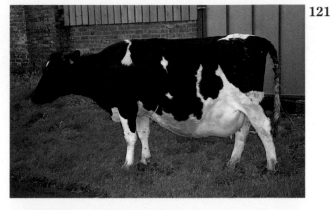

Infected ear tag

Infection of an ear tag occurs when insufficient space is allowed for growth of the ear margin, or when the tag is inserted too close to the ear base. In **122** granulation tissue and a wet, purulent exudate have developed around the tag. Such areas are painful and subject to myiasis. The tag must be removed.

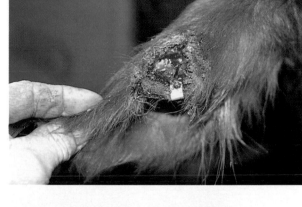

Ear necrosis from frostbite

The tips of both ears of the Limousin cow (**123**) are missing: the cause was neonatal frostbite. Septicaemia, e.g., associated with peracute salmonellosis (**50**), fescue toxicity (**401**) and ergot poisoning (**402**), can produce similar changes in the extremities. Scrotal frostbite is illustrated in **528**.

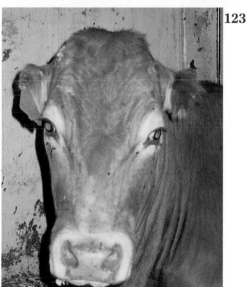

Skin necrosis following caustic dehorning paste

Excessive use of caustic dehorning paste produced the scab-covered skin slough extending from the horn bud towards the eye of this Limousin calf (**124**).

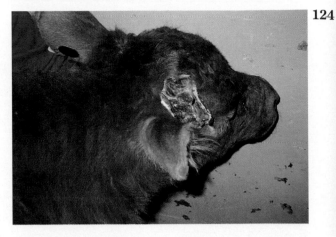

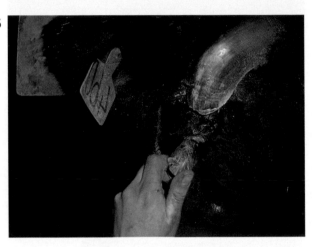

Ingrowing horn

Due to damage earlier in life, abnormal horn growth has occurred (**125**). The horn tip has penetrated through the skin into the underlying dermis, producing a painful, festering wound, which could develop secondary myiasis. Other cases develop as a result of apparently normal horn growth in older cattle.

Tail constriction caused by marker tape

In this cow (**126**) the constricting tape has been removed from the tail, revealing ischaemic necrosis and ulceration. In more advanced cases the tail tip may slough.

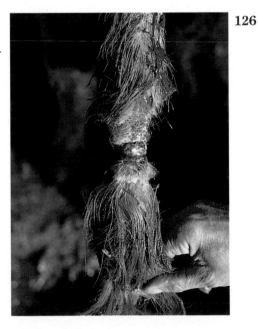

Faecolith

Faecoliths (hard accumulations of dry faeces on the tail, developing during bouts of diarrhoea) can occur spontaneously, or may develop around tail marker tape. As the faecal mass dries, it contracts, constricts the blood flow and produces swelling and ulceration, as seen on the left of the faecolith in **127**. When removed, the full extent of the ischaemic necrosis is apparent (**128**). The tail tip eventually sloughed.

127

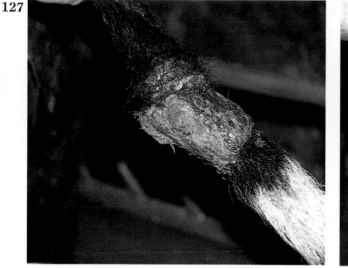

128

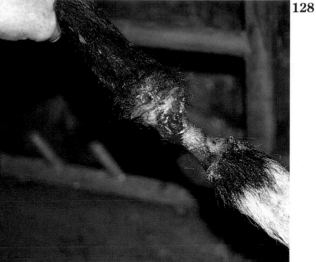

·Traumatic arterial haemorrhage from carpus

Relatively small injuries at the carpus can cause persistent haemorrhage, as in this Friesian cow (**129**).

129

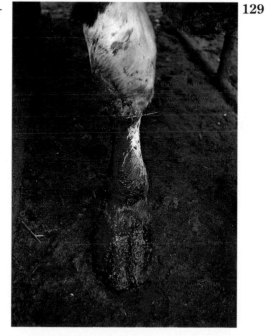

4 Alimentary disorders

Introduction

Chapter 4 illustrates those conditions with primary alimentary signs. It excludes congenital (e.g., cleft palate) and acquired neonatal conditions (e.g., calfhood enteritis). The first section comprises infectious and contagious diseases: bovine virus diarrhoea/mucosal disease (BVD/MD) complex, vesicular stomatitis, papular stomatitis (all of which have rather similar gross features), and paratuberculosis. The second section covers the alimentary parasitic conditions: ostertagiasis, and small and large intestinal parasitism (for coccidiosis, see **54** & **55**). The remaining conditions are listed by anatomical site (oral cavity to anus), irrespective of their traumatic, nutritional or other aetiology.

Viral diseases

Three viral diseases present problems clinically in differential diagnosis: bovine virus diarrhoea/mucosal disease (BVD/MD), vesicular stomatitis, and bovine papular stomatitis. In some regions, further differential diagnosis from foot-and-mouth disease and rinderpest may be necessary (see **629–640**). The pathogenicity and economic importance of these vesicular viral diseases vary greatly. Accurate differentiation is essential and usually depends on laboratory studies.

Bovine virus diarrhoea/mucosal disease (BVD/MD)

BVD/MD is a major viral disease worldwide. Congenital defects such as cerebellar hypoplasia may develop in the progeny of females infected during early pregnancy. BVD/MD causes diarrhoea and unthriftiness in young cattle. Erosive stomatitis and rhinitis occur, together with similar lesions on other mucous membranes.

In utero infection in the first trimester resulted in the birth of the Friesian calf in **130**. Though alert, it was unable to stand, and cerebellar hypoplasia was confirmed at postmortem examination. **131** shows a normal brain (left) and the affected brain.

130
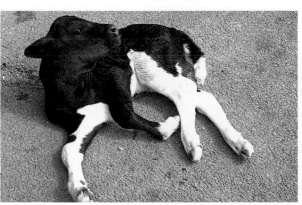

131
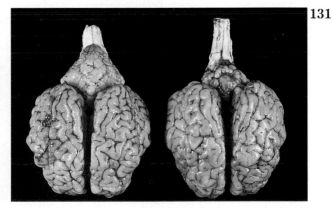

Early erosions of the gums and lips are seen in the calf in **132**. Two types of hard and soft palate changes are also illustrated: the first case (**133**) has numerous erosive lesions over the entire hard palate; the second (**134**) has more discrete, circular lesions suggestive of a secondary infection, with a raised edge primarily on the soft palate.

The oesophagus may have patchy, linear areas of haemorrhage, oedema and erosions (**135**). Secondary bacterial infection of the lesion can involve the caudal pharynx and rima glottidis (**136**). Necrosis and abscessation surround the epiglottis. The laryngeal mucosa is also haemorrhagic. Pus lies between the arytenoids, making respiratory efforts extremely difficult and painful.

132

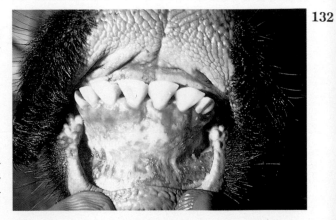

133

134

135

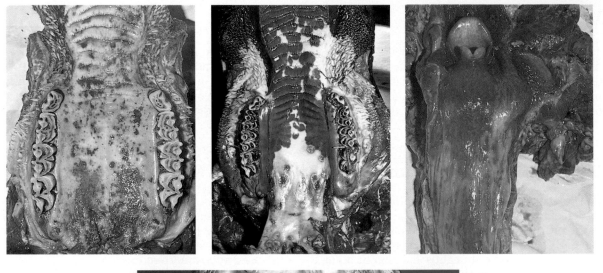

136

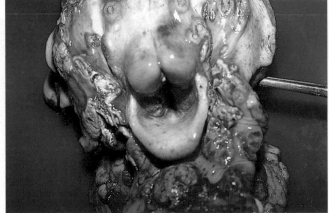

Erosions may be seen on the oedematous and hyperaemic edges of the abomasal rugae (**137**). Small intestinal erosions can lead to mucosal sloughing and the production of casts that pack the intestinal lumen (**138**). Secondary bacterial infection is probably responsible for the enlarged nodes. Erosions are also common in the interdigital cleft.

The two cattle in **139** are both 18 months old. The nearer heifer, with an abnormal, rust-coloured coat, is stunted as a result of chronic, persistent infection (antigen positive, antibody negative) due to maternal infection with BVD virus acquired in early pregnancy. Many of the mucosal changes are so severe as to leave the chronic, persistent infective case emaciated (as in the crossbred animal in **140**) and a constant source of infection to susceptible contact cattle.

137

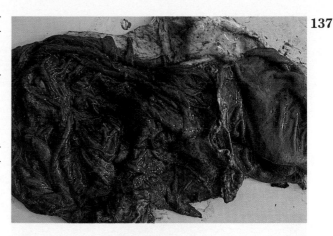

138

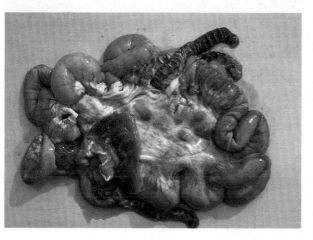

139

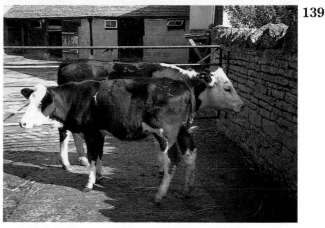

140

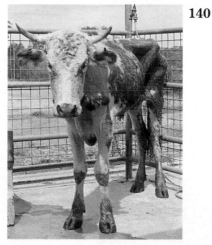

Vesicular stomatitis

The Charolais calf shows blanched areas on the rugae of the hard palate, dental pad and gums (**141**). These pale areas are vesicles that rupture after some days (**142**). Secondary infection is rare. Vesicular stomatitis has only been confirmed in North and South America. The cause is a rhabdovirus, probably spread by insect vectors. Many animals may be simultaneously affect-ed on one farm, showing excessive salivation, together with oral and possibly teat lesions. Teat lesions (**604**) in vesicular stomatitis can cause problems with milking. *Differential diagnosis*: foot-and-mouth disease (**629–633**) and papular bovine stomatitis (**143 & 144**).

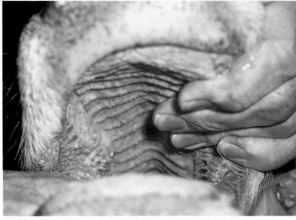

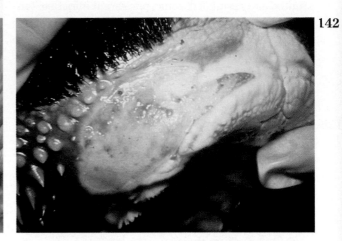

Bovine papular stomatitis (BPS)

Shallow papules and vesicles are seen on the muzzle, hard palate and gums of these young cattle (**143 & 144**). Papules develop a distinct roughened centre that sometimes expands to merge with adjacent vesicles. Teats are not affected. Immature cattle are usually involved and recovery is rapid. Systemic effects of this poxvirus (paravaccinia) are rare. *Differential diagnosis*: foot-and-mouth disease and vesicular stomatitis.

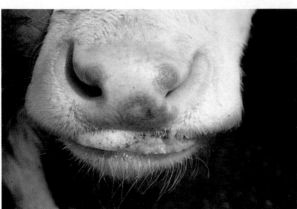

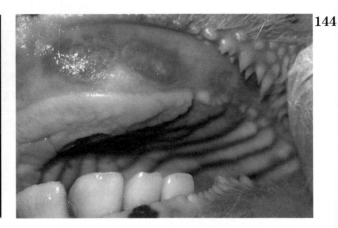

Johne's disease (paratuberculosis)

Johne's disease causes progressive weight loss, leading to eventual emaciation, although animals may remain alert and continue to eat. This chronic wasting disease, characterised by a profuse, watery diarrhoea and caused by *Mycobacterium paratuberculosis*, is seen in an eight-year-old Santa Gertrudis cow (**145**). When compared with normal ileum (**146**), the mucosa in a clinically overt case (A) shows numerous, thick,

transverse rugae that cannot be smoothed out by stretching. Local intestinal lymph nodes are usually enlarged and pale, and may contain granulomatous areas. The usual age range is 3–9 years for the onset of clinical signs, which may be insidious. Infection is introduced into healthy herds by subclinical carriers. Oral ingestion of infective organisms by young calves then takes place.

145

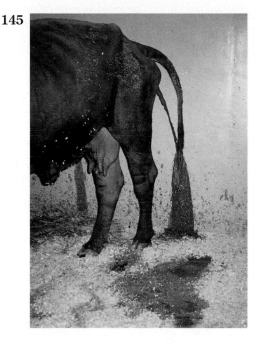

146

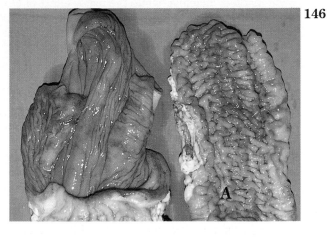

Winter dysentery (winter diarrhoea)

A watery diarrhoea (**147**) lasting about three days, winter dysentery causes a sporadic problem in adult dairy cattle. The aetiology is uncertain, although coronavirus has recently been implicated. Spontaneous recovery usually takes place after a few days. *Differential diagnosis:* Johne's disease (**145**), rumenitis or overeating (**175**).

147

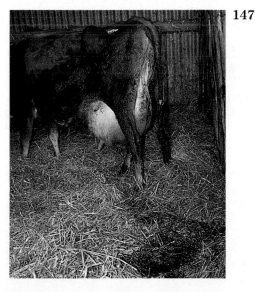

Gastrointestinal parasitism

The major gastrointestinal parasites of cattle are the stomach (abomasal) worms *Haemonchus placei* (barber's pole worm or large stomach worm, 18–30 mm long male), *Ostertagia ostertagi* (medium or brown stomach worm, 6–9 mm long), and *Trichostrongylus axei* (small stomach worm, 5 mm long). In tropical regions, other species, e.g., *Mecistocirrus digitatus*, are significant. Severe infestations of *Haemonchus* can cause marked anaemia, while the major effect of *Ostertagia* and *Trichostrongylus* is a severe, protein-losing enteropathy, characterised by a profuse, watery diarrhoea. All three species have the facility for their embryonated eggs or infective larvae to survive in faeces for weeks or months at lower temperatures or in drought conditions, until a favourable environment returns.

Of the three species, *Ostertagia ostertagi* is overall the most pathogenic and economically important in most temperate regions of the world, including Great Britain and much of the USA. As with most gastrointestinal parasites, the most severe effects are seen in growing animals. Nevertheless, it can be a devastatingly debilitating disease in susceptible adults.

Ostertagiasis

Cattle are most commonly affected with a chronic, persistent diarrhoea and weight loss during their first season at pasture. Type I disease caused by *Ostertagia ostertagi* results from the ingestion of large numbers of L_3 larvae from herbage, starting 3–6 weeks before the onset of clinical signs. Small nodules that are 1–2mm in diameter are present on and between the abomasal folds on the mucosal surface (**148**). In severe cases a 'Morocco leather' or 'cobblestoned' appearance is evident (**149**). Higher magnification of a severe case shows the thickened ridges and the white worms (**150**). Weight loss, chronic diarrhoea and tenesmus are seen in an older Charolais heifer (**151**) with Type II disease, which occurs when many dormant larvae (early L_4) emerge from the abomasal glands.

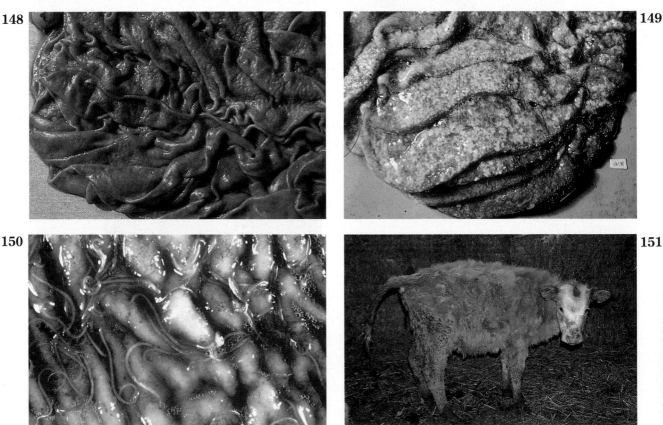

Oesophagostomum infection

152 shows the serosal surface of the large intestine. Numerous caseated and calcified nodules indicate the presence of *Oesophagostomum radiatum* (nodular worm) in an older, resistant animal. Clinical signs tend to be much less severe than with *Ostertagia*. Heavy worm burdens in calves cause anorexia, severe, dark diarrhoea and weight loss. In older animals the nodules affect gut motility. These nodules can be palpated *per rectum*. The worms measure 12–15 mm long and the head is angled to the body.

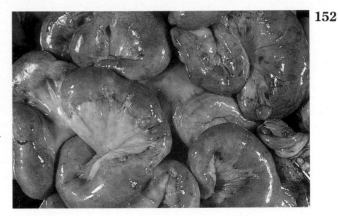

152

Dental problems

Excessive incisor wear

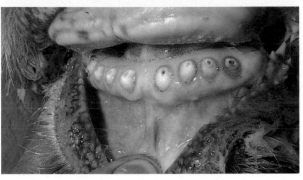

153

Cattle rarely have dental problems leading to clinical disease. Occasionally, when the temporary incisors are being replaced by the permanent dentition, 2–3-year-old heifers show difficulty in prehension. Diets leading to excessive incisor wear may cause progressive weight loss (**153**). The crowns have almost disappeared, resulting in impairment of the animal's foraging ability.

Fluorosis

Fluorosis (**154**) leads to mottling and excessive wear of temporary teeth during their development (see also Chapter 13, **727** & **728**).

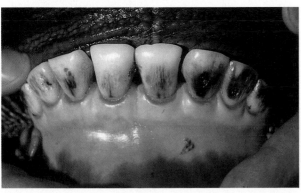

154

Dental discolouration

Fluorine-induced discolouration should be differentiated from the staining caused by ingestion of some forms of grass silage, as shown in **155**.

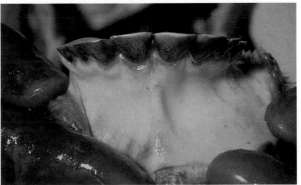

155

Irregular molar wear

Irregular molar wear can sometimes cause masticatory problems. When eating or ruminating, this eight-year-old bull (**156**) occasionally kept the jaws apart as a result of 'locking' the overgrown lingual edge of the upper molars and premolars against the buccal edge of the mandibular cheek teeth. The length of the bilaterally symmetrical overgrowth was about 1 cm. **156** shows the typical open 'locked' position.

Mandibular fracture

Mandibular fractures usually result from iatrogenic trauma. In the mature Friesian cow (**157**) with the symphysial fracture, the left central incisor was lost. There was little separation of the two halves of the mandible. A considerable quantity of saliva is being lost. In this case the cause of the fracture was unknown. Full recovery occurred without treatment.

Discrete swellings of the head

Actinobacillosis, actinomycosis and local abscessation related to *Actinomyces pyogenes* can present similar clinical features in some cattle. Typically, however, actinobacillosis affects the soft tissues, especially the tongue, while actinomycosis involves bone. Abscessation related to tooth root infection is rare in cattle.

Actinobacillosis ('wooden tongue')

Actinobacillus lignieresi preferentially colonises the soft tissues of the head, especially the tongue. It typically causes a localised, firm swelling of the dorsum, as in this dairy cow (**158**). Occasionally, the tongue has nodules over much of the surface except the tip (**159**). Other parts of the head, such as the nares (**160**) or facial skin, are sometimes alone affected. Rarely, other areas of the body (e.g., the limbs, **161**) develop cutaneous actinobacillosis. Skin infection usually follows trauma and exposure to a concentrated infective dose of organisms. Such massive lesions are particularly liable to bleed and ulcerate. Most cases tend to occur in mature cattle of dairy breeds.

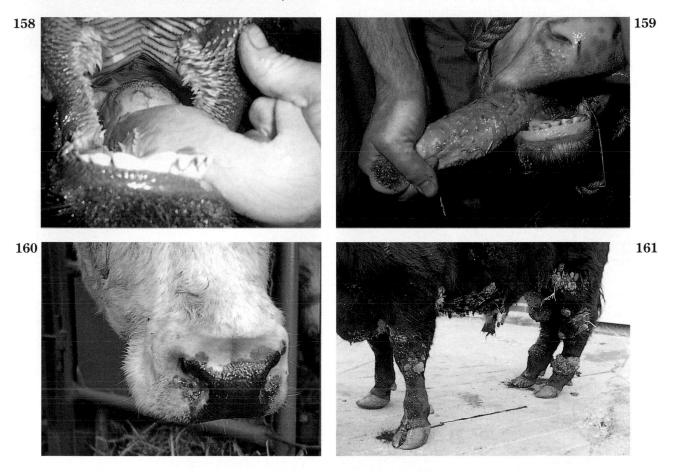

158 **159** **160** **161**

Actinomycosis ('lumpy jaw')

Actinomycosis (*Actinomyces bovis*) causes a rarefying periostitis of the maxilla and the mandible, with a surrounding soft tissue reaction. The Guernsey cow in **162** has a right maxillary swelling and several granulomatous masses have broken through the skin. The cow experienced no apparent interference with mastication for 18 months after the swelling was first seen. The crossbred Hereford cow with 'lumpy jaw' (**163**) had moderate difficulty in chewing. A large, fist-sized, proliferating mass lies over the angle of the mandible. Despite secondary infection, body condition remained good. Dysphagia is usually due to malalignment of molar teeth. A lateral radiograph (**164**) of a two-year-old heifer with mandibular actinomycosis (in considerable discomfort and rapidly losing weight) shows massive periosteal new bone formation (A) and cavitation (B). *Differential diagnosis*: mandibular abscess (**169**) and actinobacillosis (**158–161**).

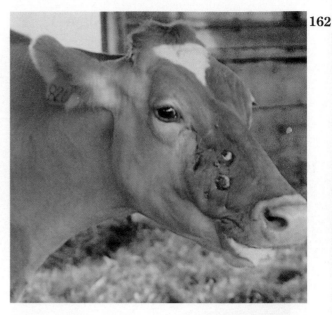

162

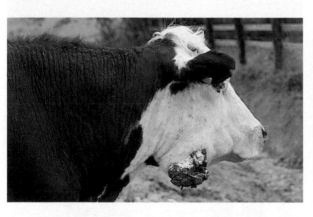

163

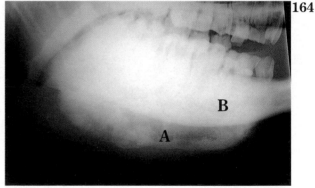

164

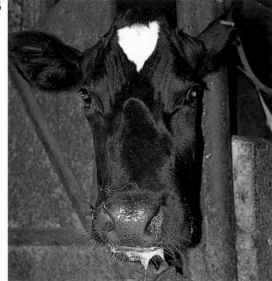

165

Malignant oedema (necrotic cellulitis)

Malignant oedema is caused by *Clostridium septicum* and results from contaminated wounds in any superficial part of the body. In this cow (**165**), infection entered the masseter area of the right cheek to cause a rapidly enlarging and unilateral soft tissue swelling, especially obvious around the right nostril. There was pronounced salivation. The brisket is enlarged with oedematous fluid (**166**). Despite prompt, prolonged antibiotic therapy, infection spread to the forelegs and, as in many cases, was fatal. Gas formation is rare. *Differential diagnosis*: cutaneous urticaria (blaine) (**68**) and abscessation (**169**).

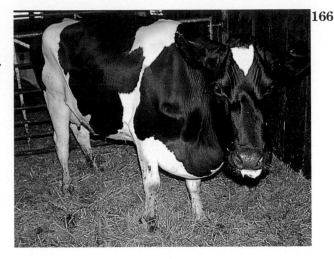

166

Alveolar periostitis (*Cara inchada,* 'swollen face')

Alveolar periostitis is a major problem in some parts of South America, such as Brazil. Periodontal disease affects the sockets of the upper premolars and molars in calves following a severe gingivitis and secondary bacterial infection (*Actinomyces pyogenes* and *Bacteroides melaninogenicus*). The first sign is uni- or bilateral swelling of the cheek as a result of impaction by pasture grass. Postmortem examination reveals loss or marked displacement of several temporary teeth, particularly premolars two and three, and a massive periosteal and osteolytic reaction in the related maxilla (**167** & **168**). On pastures of guinea grass (*Panicum*

maximum), which causes traumatic damage to the gingiva, the condition leads to malnutrition and sometimes death. The 18-month-old mixed Zebu steer from the Mato Grosso (**167**) has lost the right second and third upper premolars (A) and the left second premolar (B). Loss of the surrounding cement has led to deep pockets on the labial side of the right arcade (C). The steer was severely emaciated. **168** shows a similar type of animal. A striking, chronic, ossifying periostitis affects the region around the roots of P2 and P3, explaining the likelihood of tooth loss.

167

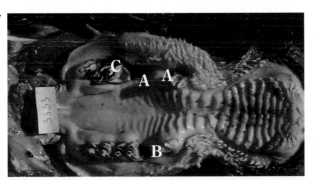

168

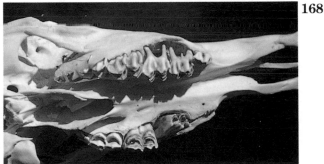

Submandibular abscess

Caused by *Actinomyces pyogenes*, a smooth and localised soft tissue swelling, discharging pus, lies over the horizontal ramus of the left mandible (**169**). It developed rapidly over three weeks and resolved slowly. *Differential diagnosis*: actinomycosis (**162**) and fracture of the mandible (**157**).

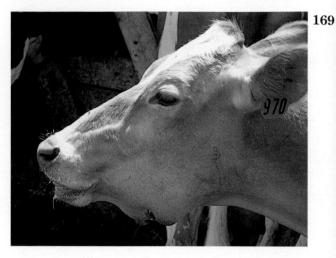

169

Pharyngeal and retropharyngeal swellings

Pharyngeal and retropharyngeal swellings can range from being innocuous to rapidly fatal. Careful external and oral/pharyngeal examination is essential. A swelling may be indicative of systemic disease elsewhere, such as right heart failure manifested as submandibular and retropharyngeal oedema (**258**). The swelling may involve retropharyngeal and parotid lymph nodes in a neoplastic reaction (**691**). Severe reactions in the submucosal tissues of the pharynx, with potentially dire consequences to the airway and possibly death, can result either from the introduction of a small amount of irritant material (e.g., poloxalene) through an accidental puncture wound, or from extensive lacerations to the pharyngeal wall, which then fails to heal rapidly.

Drenching gun injury

Perforation of the pharyngeal wall by a drenching gun caused a septic cellulitis leading to the grossly enlarged parotid region (**170**). One consequence of this cellulitis was a malodorous, purulent nasal and oral discharge. The heifer was pyrexic and anorexic. Post-mortem examination of another case (**171**) revealed masses of inspissated pus beneath the pharyngeal and laryngeal mucosae, which had caused respiratory embarrassment (inspiratory stridor). Note the congestion of the mucosal surface of the epiglottis.

170

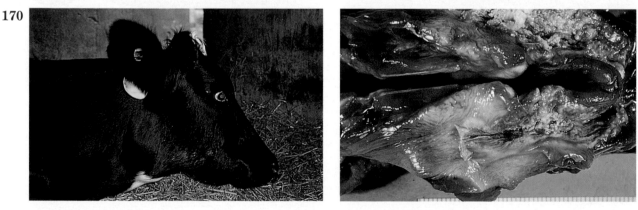

171

Retropharyngeal abscess

A discrete and relatively painless fluctuating, tennis ball-sized mass lies in the retropharyngeal region (**172**). The spread of infection (compare **170**) was limited by the development of a fibrous capsule. Abscessation in this region is often a result of accidental pharyngeal damage from drenching or balling guns, probangs or other rigid instruments.

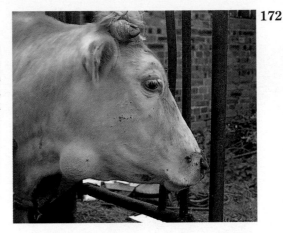
172

Oesophageal obstruction

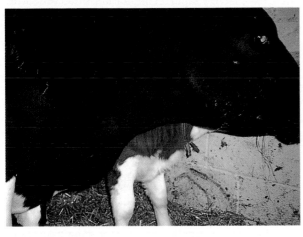
73

A potato is lodged two-thirds of the way down the cervical oesophagus (**173**). The animal was uncomfortable and drooling as a result of its inability to swallow saliva. Since eructation was impeded, it also had rumen tympany. Common sites of oesophageal obstruction are just dorsal to the larynx and at the thoracic inlet. In cattle, oesophageal foreign bodies tend to be solid objects, such as hedge apples, large portions of turnips or beets, or ears of corn (maize). Other suspicious signs of oesophageal obstruction include extension of the head and neck, dyspnoea, occasional coughing, and chewing movements. A cervical oesophageal foreign body is readily palpated externally. *Differential diagnosis*: rabies (**478–482**) and acute rumenitis (**175–179**).

Megaoesophagus

The entire cervical oesophagus (**174**) is grossly distended (about 5–6 cm in diameter). Contrast radiography revealed a similar distension of most of the thoracic oesophagus. The abnormality had been first observed at one year of age. Clinical signs included frequent regurgitation. The 15-month-old Charolais heifer was observed for one year and almost completely recovered. Megaoesophagus is rare and, although usually congenital, this case was probably secondary to a systemic infection.

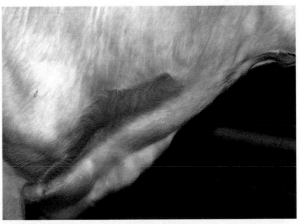
174

Rumenitis and omasitis of dietary origin

175

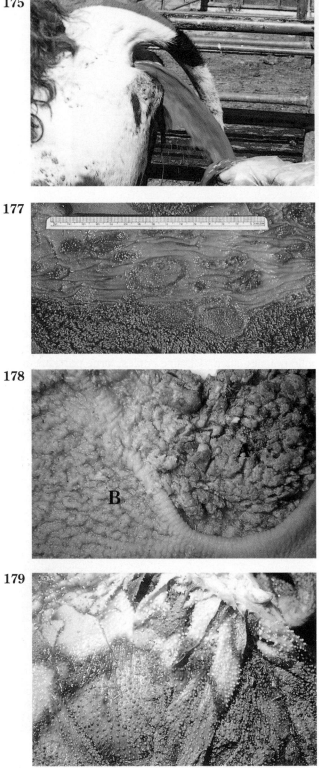

176

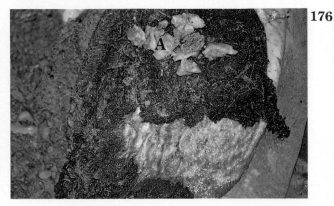

177

178

179

Over-eating of grain (corn), resulting in excessively rapid fermentation, can lead to a chemical rumenitis, laminitis (**326**) and severe metabolic acidosis as a result of excessively rapid fermentation. Affected cattle are very dull, weak, ataxic or recumbent. A light-coloured diarrhoea containing grain particles may be seen (**175**). Ruminal pH is usually very acidic (pH < 5). **176** shows areas of sloughed ruminal epithelium and intense serosal haemorrhage in a 10-month-old Simmental bull which died 24 hours after access to fodder beet. Whole fragments of undigested fodder beet are clearly visible (A). Four to six days after a grain overload, a mycotic or fusobacterial rumenitis may be seen (**177**), comprising sharply defined, oval lesions that are often red or dark, and relatively thick. A close-up view of a more chronic rumenitis (**178**) shows a rumen fold separating the disorganised and necrotic rumenal papillae (A) from more normal papillae (B). In rumenitis colonised by *Fusobacteria* and fungi, healing eventually occurs after sloughing of the necrotic layers, contraction of the ulcer, and peripheral epithelial regeneration, resulting in stellate scar formation. The omasum in **179** shows a fungal infection (most likely due to *Aspergillus* species) following the accidental ingestion of mouldy feed, e.g., cereals or beans. Changes are most common in the ruminoreticulum (**177**) and the occurrence in the omasum is rare.

Rumen tympany ('bloat')

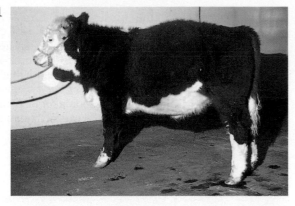

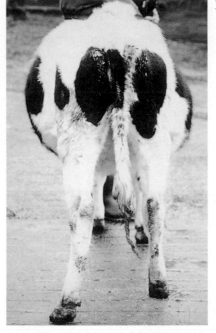

The Holstein heifer in **180** has an obvious distension of the left paralumbar fossa. The swelling may extend above the level of the lumbar spine, as seen in the Hereford steer (**181**). Both animals had a gaseous as opposed to a foamy (or frothy) bloat. Possible causes include oesophageal obstruction (**173**), an oesophageal groove mass (**182**) and rumenal atony. (For bloat in a calf, see **56**).

Ruminal neoplasia

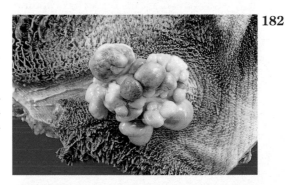

This pedunculated mass (**182**) is a benign papilloma. Lying at the proximal end of the oesophageal groove, it caused partial obstruction of the lower oesophageal sphincter, resulting in an intermittent ruminal tympany. Diagnosis of ruminal neoplasia requires an exploratory rumenotomy to differentiate neoplasia from actinobacillosis of the oesophageal groove, chronic reticulitis or reticular wall abscessation. (See **184** for another ruminoreticular neoplasm (fibroma).)

Abdominal pain

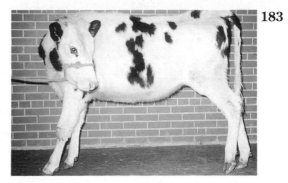

In comparison with the horse, the signs of pain seen in this heifer (**183**) are uncommon. The forefeet are placed further forward than normal, presumably in an attempt to reduce tension on the abdominal viscera. The head is turned towards the flank. The tail is slightly elevated (indicative of tenesmus) and the heifer is kicking at the belly with a hind foot. The stance suggests an intestinal problem. Posterior abdominal pain can result in tenesmus that may not necessarily reflect an alimentary origin, for example, babesiosis, **655–660**), cystitis (**505**) or urethritis (**499**).

Traumatic reticulitis

This section of the reticular wall illustrates the typical wires (**184**) that may perforate the wall to cause a localised or generalised peritonitis (**205** & **206**), hepatic abscessation (**216**), or may travel cranially to produce a septic pericarditis (**263** & **264**). An incidental abnormality in this reticulum (**184**) was a discrete pedunculated fibroma (A). Cattle with acute reticuloperitonitis are pyrexic and grunt during reticular movements.

Animals suffering from traumatic reticulitis may rapidly become dehydrated, one sign of which is obvious skin 'tenting' (**185**): the skin fold remains for 3–10 seconds or more (indicating approximately 6–12% dehydration). They appear dejected, have an arched back, sunken eyes (**186**) as a result of the dehydration, weight loss, and an empty flank and 'tucked up' belly due to lack of rumen fill (**187**). *Differential diagnosis*: left (**197**) or right (**199**) displaced abomasum, abomasal ulceration with perforation (**192**), caecal dilatation (**201**) and bacterial endocarditis (**262**).

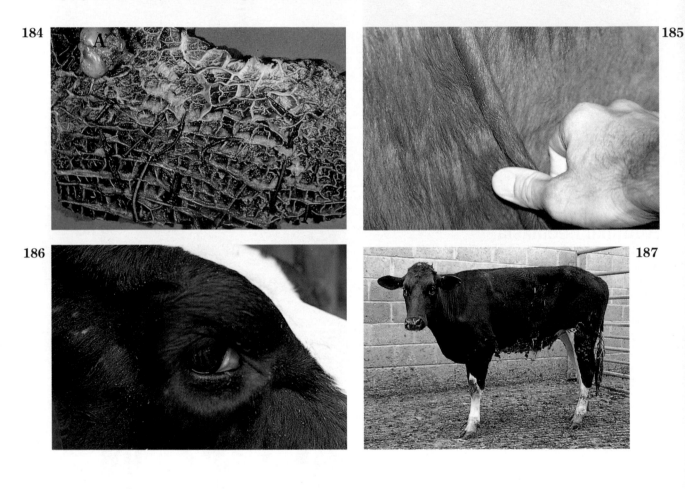

Forestomach or abomasal obstructive syndrome (vagal indigestion, Hoflund syndrome)

The silhouette of the abdominal wall shows a massive, left-sided swelling due to an accumulation of fluid, primarily in the ruminoreticulum (**188**). After pumping out 90 litres, the flanks became almost symmetrical (**189**). The distension is characteristically in the upper left and lower right flanks, resulting in the so-called 'ten-to-four' appearance. **190** is a typical example. The cause of vagal indigestion, or Hoflund syndrome, is a functional disturbance of the normal motility of the forestomachs or the abomasum, or of all compartments.

Ruminoreticular distension that results from vagal dysfunction due to reticuloperitonitis is the most common form (**190**). Severe ruminal distension is most marked in the left sublumbar fossa and low down in the right flank (so-called 'papple-shaped', i.e., pear x apple).

Discrete omasal obstruction (as opposed to secondary abomasal obstruction) due to reticuloperitonitis is rare. When compared with **188**, the abdominal silhouette of the two-year-old Holstein bull in **191** is similarly asymmetrical, showing distension of the upper left (ruminoreticulum) and lower right (omasum, and to a lesser extent ruminoreticulum) flanks. The cause of the omasal obstruction was secondary impaction due to a reticular wall abscess (foreign body:wire) and a localised reticuloperitonitis. Mechanical causes, such as neoplastic infiltration near the pylorus, can lead to similar effects. Diagnosis depends on exploratory laparotomy. *Differential diagnosis*: chronic traumatic reticulitis, peritonitis, rumen tympany, abomasal impaction and obstruction of the reticulo-omasal orifice.

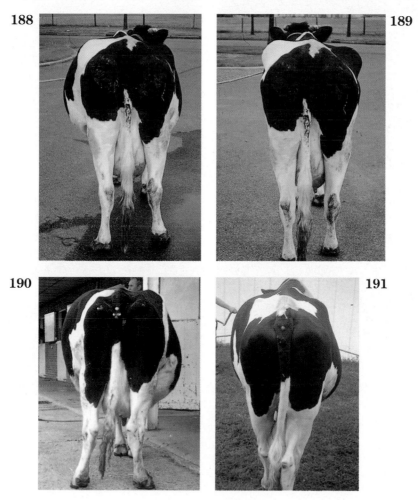

188

189

190

191

Abomasal ulceration

Abomasal ulceration occurs in mature dairy and beef cattle and in calves. Some cases in adults are the result of primary diseases such as infiltrative lymphosarcoma, and systemic infections such as BVD and malignant bovine catarrh. In high-yielding dairy cows, ulcers are usually associated with stress and high concentrate rations. Multiple abomasal ulcers may occur in calves (**52**). There are four types of ulcer, Type I being that which causes no clinically apparent disease. Type II is a bleeding ulcer that, if persistent, results in progressive anaemia. Types III and IV cause an acute localised or generalised peritonitis with signs of pain and Type IV is almost always fatal.

The Guernsey cow in **192** had abdominal pain due to a Type III (perforating) abomasal ulcer causing a localised peritonitis, evident in the depressed appearance, arched posture and forward-placed hindlegs. She passed black, tarry faeces containing much digested blood (**193**). Cows sometimes die following severe blood loss into the abomasal lumen. Postmortem examination (**194**) reveals numerous ulcers, several filled with blood (A), and a diffuse abomasitis. The pathology is similar to that of the calfhood disease (**51–53**), with localised or generalised peritonitis as possible sequelae. Healing abomasal ulcers (**195**) show scar tissue causing contraction of the abomasal wall in a stellate pattern. Some bleeding was still occuring. *Differential diagnosis*: traumatic reticulitis, abomasitis and abomasal lymphoma (lymphosarcoma) (**196**).

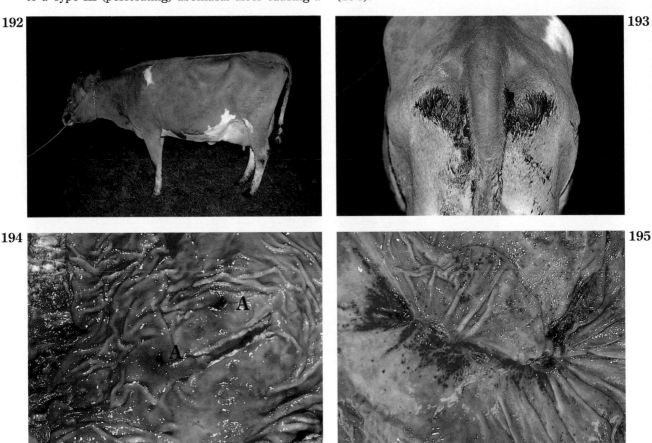

192 193 194 195

Abomasal lymphoma

This specimen from an old Holstein cow shows thickened and irregular abomasal rugae as a result of lymphoma infiltration (**196**). The discrete, dark, punched-out areas are ulcers, indicating that the two conditions can occur together. Neoplastic infiltration was widespread.

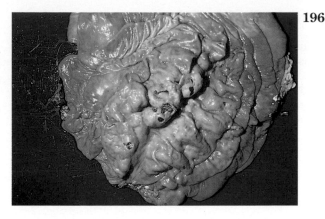

Abomasal surgical conditions

In areas of intensive management, left and, to a lesser extent, right abomasal displacements are common conditions in dairy cattle. Right abomasal torsion can be a serious secondary complication of right abomasal displacement. Most cases of mechanical displacement of this type occur in high yielding cows in early lactation, and are preceded by a period of abomasal hypotony or atony. A proportion have secondary problems such as ketosis, metritis or mastitis.

Left displaced abomasum

The displaced abomasum is situated almost entirely beneath the rib cage on the left, where it can be detected by percussion and auscultation. The caudal, dorsal portion may extend behind the last rib to form a palpable, soft swelling which can then be distinguished from the underlying rumen in the paralumbar fossa. In **197** the abomasum (A) may be seen through a left paralumbar vertical incision lying between the cranial edge of the incision and the spleen (B), which is cranial to the visible portion (C) of rumen wall. Chronic and persistent left abomasal displacement results in a slow loss of condition due to partial inappetence. The bulge (A) of the abomasum may then become more obvious in the left flank (**198**).

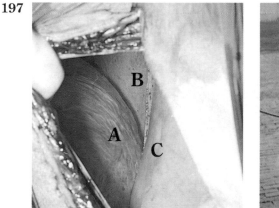

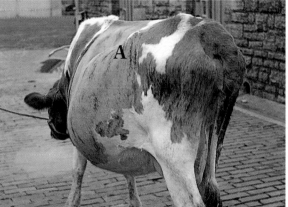

Right displaced abomasum

In this Guernsey cow (**199**) the distended abomasum is seen through a vertical right flank paralumbar incision about 7 cm caudal to the last rib. The remainder of the abomasum is located medial to the costal arch. The greater omentum containing the descending duodenum (A), is seen caudal to the abomasal swelling.

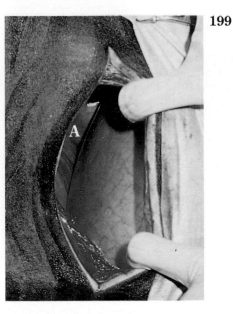

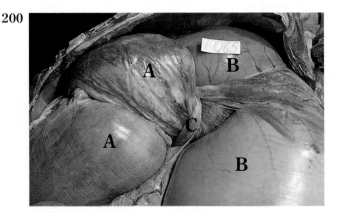

Abomasal torsion

A postmortem specimen (**200**) of the abomasum (A), ruminoreticulum (B) and duodenum (C) shows a complex torsion of both the abomasum and omasum. Typically, the cow was found in extreme shock. The abomasal fluid volume exceeded 90 litres (normal volume: 10–20 litres).

Caecal torsion

Following caecal displacement and distension, this Holstein cow developed an acute (painful) abdomen within 48 hours. The enlarged caecum was appreciable on rectal palpation. The caecal apex has been prolapsed through a dorsal and caudal right flank laparotomy incision (**201**), but most of the caecum still lies within the abdominal cavity. The peritoneal surface is slightly congested. Many cases of simple caecal dilatation are asymptomatic.

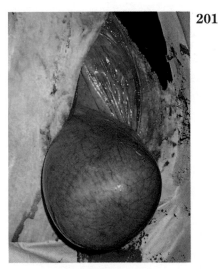

Jejunal torsion and intussusception ('twisted gut')

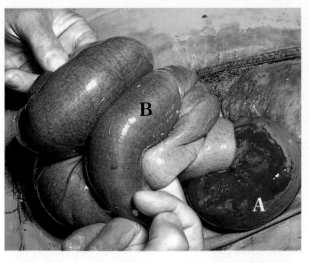

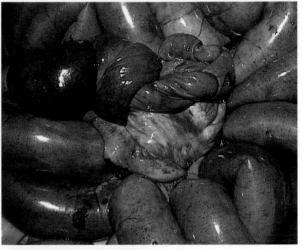

Intussusception is the most common cause of small intestinal obstruction in cattle. Occurring at any age, it initially causes severe abdominal pain. In **202** the darker loop of small intestine (A), showing marked congestion and subserosal haemorrhage, particularly on the mesenteric border, is the segment of bowel through which the intussusception has passed. Dilated proximal intestine is seen at B. The point of invagination of the intussusception is not visible in this picture, it being tightly knotted deeply below the position of the fingers.

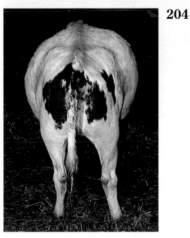

Another case (**203**) illustrates the severe and complex nature of bovine intussusception. The site of intussusception is clearly visible (A). Several jejunal loops have undergone torsion. Affected animals often have a grossly distended abdomen (**204**) due to fluid accumulation in the prestenotic small intestinal loops, abomasum and ruminoreticulum.

Peritonitis

Inflammation of the peritoneal cavity may be localised or generalised, acute or chronic. In active disease, guarding of the abdomen results in a stiff gait (see p. 66). The bovine peritoneum and greater omentum have a remarkable facility to wall off leaks of bowel contents and localised areas of abscessation. This process oftens results in few or no complications in the cranial part of the abdomen. Adhesions developing in the caudal part can cause progressive bowel obstruction. In **205** the visceral and parietal peritoneum (rumen, jejunum and greater omentum) is covered

with a fibrinous and purulent exudate, typical of early generalised peritonitis. The changes are more advanced and chronic in another case (**206**), resulting from septic reticuloperitonitis (see also **184**).

Other common causes of peritonitis are perforated abomasal ulcers, either in calfhood (**53**) or in adult life (**194**), and rupture of the small intestine following uncorrected intussusception or small intestinal torsion. Neonatal peritonitis may occur following the rupture of a distended small intestine proximal to an atretic bowel (**17**).

205

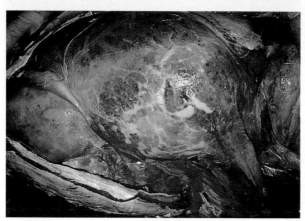

206

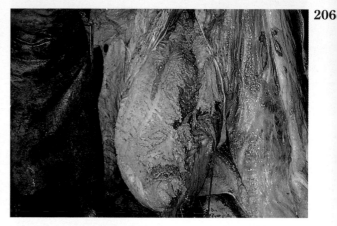

Ascites

As with peritonitis, ascites results in an accumulation of free fluid in the abdominal cavity, eventually causing a pear-shaped silhouette (**207**). Ascitic fluid is serous or oedematous in nature and is usually sterile. This old Galloway cow had hepatic cirrhosis resulting from chronic severe fascioliasis. Compare intestinal obstruction (**204**).

207

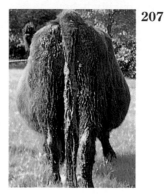

Hepatic diseases

Clinical signs of liver disease are variable and relate to the wide range of functions carried out by the liver These include bile production, synthesis of specific plasma components, detoxification, storage, and a variety of metabolic processes.

The large functional reserve of the liver results in the signs of disease usually becoming evident only when hepatic damage is extensive. There are few characteristic signs of malfunction and diagnosis often presents a major challenge to the clinician. Several specific diseases of the liver cause reduced weight gain and slaughterhouse condemnation of the liver

(abscessation, fluke infestation). Ancillary diagnostic aids include enzyme estimation (SDH, GDH, GGT) and percutaneous hepatic biopsy.

Examples of the hepatic diseases illustrated below include necrotic hepatitis caused by *Clostridium haemolyticum* (*C. novyi* or *C. oedematiens*), hepatic abscessation secondary to rumenitis, and fascioliasis resulting from severe parasitism. Although not specifically involving the liver, other forms of fluke are also included in this section. Fatty liver syndrome produced by ill-defined nutritional and metabolic imbalance is described in Chapter 9 (**458**).

Fascioliasis

The liver becomes fibrotic with enlargement, the bile ducts become grossly thickened, and mature *Fasciola hepatica* flukes occupy the lumen (**208** & **209**). The walls may eventually become calcified. The visceral surface becomes irregular and granular in appearance.

The associated fat in ligamentous attachments is lost, leaving little but the greyish peritoneal surface as emaciation develops. Clinical cases become hypoproteinaemic, developing ventral and submandibular oedema. Ascites (**207**) is a common result.

208

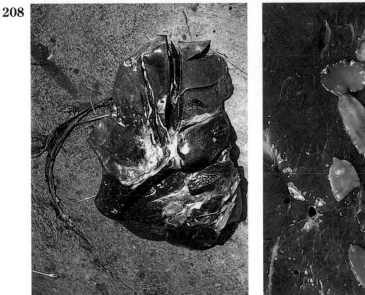

209

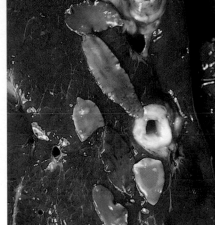

210

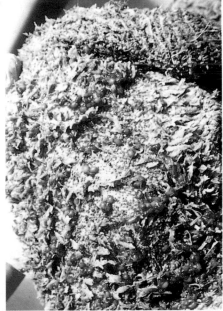

Paramphistomiasis (rumen flukes)

Even the relatively large numbers of soft, pink, pear-shaped, adult flukes seen attached to the rumen wall (**210**) cause few clinical signs, particularly in older cattle. However, immature stages attached to the duodenum may lead to unthriftiness, diarrhoea and death in young animals. Several different species of fluke including *P. cervi*, *P. microbothrium* and *P. ichikawai*, are involved. Snails act as intermediate hosts.

Schistosomiasis (blood flukes)

Eight species of *Schistosoma* have been reported throughout Africa, the Middle East and Asia. Cercariae, released into water from the intermediate snail host, penetrate the skin or mucous membranes. **211** shows a pair of elongated flukes in a blood vessel of the stretched mesentery (A), with the female lying in a longitudinal groove of the male. Flukes may be up to 30 mm long. Pathogenic species are primarily found in mesenteric blood vessels, although one species, *S. nasale*, inhabits the nasal mucosa. The major clinical signs of haemorrhagic enteritis and emaciation are seen when the spiny eggs pass through the gut wall. In the hepatic form, granulomas form around the eggs. Lesions may also be found in the liver, lungs and bladder. *S. nasale* (**212**) produces a proliferative reaction of granulomatous masses, seen in this median section through the nasal turbinate bones. The effect is chronic nasal obstruction and dyspnoea. The parasite inhabits the veins of the mucosa. *S. nasale* is a problem in the Indian subcontinent, Malaysia and the Caribbean. Diagnosis depends on demonstration of the eggs in faeces, rectal scrapings or, for *S. nasale*, nasal mucus.

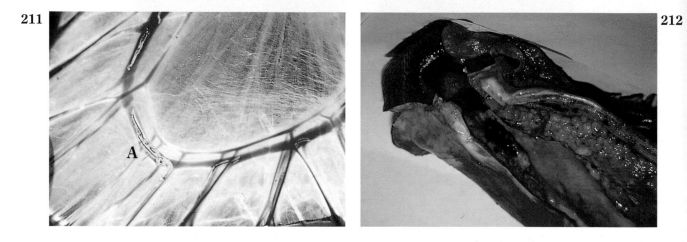

Necrotic hepatitis (bacillary haemoglobinuria, 'black disease')

Discrete, irregular, pale infarcts on the liver surface (**213**) are characteristic of this acute fatal toxaemia caused by *C. haemolyticum* (*C. novyi*). A section through another affected liver (**214**) shows a typical, large, single infarct, with scattered paler areas within it, at the margin of a liver lobe. Most frequently seen

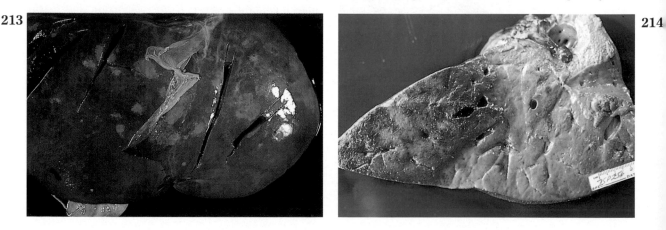

in areas of endemic fascioliasis, the larvae of *Fasciola hepatica* are the usual cause of the initial damage. The resulting lesions are then colonised by *Clostridia,* which produce a toxin causing severe depression and rapid death from toxaemia. Gross pathology may also include extensive subserosal haemorrhage, shown involving the perirenal area in **215**.

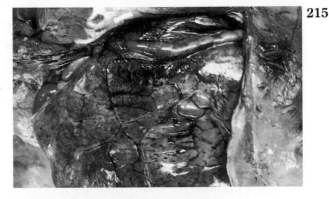

Hepatic abscessation

Hepatic abscesses are usually multiple and vary in size. In this case (**216**) a large, central abscess has ruptured to release creamy pus. The cause is usually an acute rumenitis (**176**), which is followed by a haematogenous spread to the neighbouring liver. Such abscesses usually yield *Actinomyces* on culture, although the initial hepatic colonisation is generally by *Fusobacterium necrophorum.* Fattening steers and high-yielding dairy cows are more susceptible owing to their relatively greater intake of concentrate feed. A specific complication of hepatic abscessation is posterior vena cava thrombosis (**251**) or pulmonary thromboembolism (**252**). The clinical signs include anterior abdominal pain, partial anorexia and weight loss. *Differential diagnosis:* traumatic reticulitis (**187**) and abomasal ulceration (**192**).

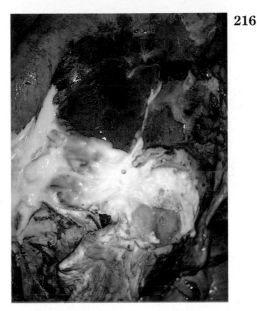

Lipomatosis (abdominal fat necrosis)

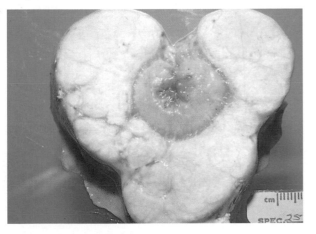

A vertical section through the pelvic cavity of an old Angus cow (**217**) shows the rectum surrounded and severely constricted by large areas of fat necrosis, which are firm, dry and caseous. Such areas, which are also called lipomata, may occur in any part of the omental, mesenteric and retroperitoneal fat. They may cause chronic progressive bowel obstruction. Although generally quite rare, lipomatosis is considered more common in mature or older Channel Island breeds. Although the aetiology is unclear, genetic factors, excessive intakes of soya beans and persistent pyrexia have been suggested.

Rectal prolapse

In **218** rectal prolapse had started 24 hours previously, primarily involving the rectal mucosa, which is still fresh and almost undamaged. The second case (**219**) had begun seven days previously and shows severe lacerations and oedema. The only undamaged area is close to the skin–mucosal junction. Rectal prolapse occurs mainly, but not exclusively, in young animals with acute, severe or chronic diarrhoea resulting in recurrent tenesmus. Two other predisposing causes of tenesmus are coccidiosis (**54**) and occasionally rabies (**479**).

218

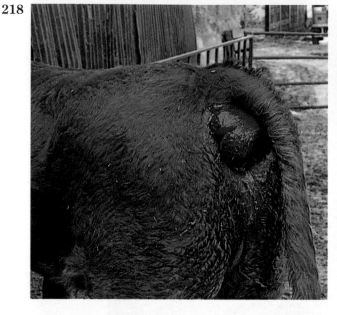

219

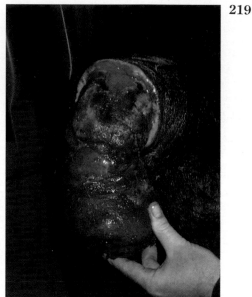

220

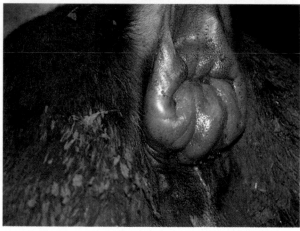

Anal oedema

Anal oedema (**220**) leading to protrusion of the recto-anal mucosa is an occasional consequence of rectal palpation.

5 Respiratory disorders

Introduction

Although respiratory diseases have a variety of causes, infectious agents predominate e.g., infectious bovine rhinotracheitis (IBR) is caused by a herpesvirus that can affect several body systems.

A second group of respiratory infections is caused by *Pasteurella*, usually following exposure of young cattle to stress (hence the alternative name for pasteurellosis, 'shipping fever'). Both *Pasteurella haemolytica* and *P. multocida* are normal inhabitants of the upper respiratory tract and in particular the tonsillar crypts. In order to permit colonisation of the lungs, stress or a primary viral infection such as bovine virus diarrhoea/mucosal disease (BVD/MD), respiratory syncytial virus (RSV) or parainfluenza type 3 P13, must compromise the defence mechanisms of the body.

A third respiratory infection, termed endemic or enzootic calf pneumonia, affects groups of young calves and is of major economic importance. Both viruses (e.g., P13, BVD, IBR, RSV, adeno- and rhinoviruses) and mycoplasmas may be primary agents, but the aetiology of many outbreaks remains uncertain, since bacterial colonisation by *Pasteurella* tends rapidly to supervene. Consequently, the primary virus infection may have been cleared by the time of postmortem examination. The role of *Chlamydia* is unclear.

Haemophilus somnus is of major importance as a cause of suppurative pneumonia (**475**), but having effects on several organ systems, it is presented as infectious thromboembolic meningoencephalitis in Chapter 9.

Respiratory diseases in young cattle are of great economic importance, since their immunity to many aetiological agents is poor and vaccination regimes therefore have severe limitations. Antibiotic therapy can be very costly, and those cattle which recover, often show poor weight gain. Contagious bovine pleuropneumonia is a problem in many developing countries, such as parts of Africa, India and China, where eradication through a slaughter policy and vaccination programmes presents major organisational problems.

Chapter 5 is divided into infectious (viral, bacterial and other agents) and non-infectious (allergic, iatrogenic, circulatory and physiological) aetiology. Where appropriate, cross-reference is made to other sections for lesions affecting other systems; for example, both calf diphtheria and laryngeal abscessation (**61–64**) are shown in the neonatal chapter, even though they sometimes occur in older animals.

Infectious bovine rhinotracheitis (IBR) ('rednose')

The common respiratory form of IBR has major clinical signs involving the nostrils (hence the alternative name of 'rednose') and the eyes. Within a group of young cattle, several individuals may be affected simultaneously with epiphora and depression. Severely affected animals, such as the crossbred neonate in **221**, are dull, somnolent, anorexic with a tucked-up belly, and have a mucopurulent nasal discharge, nasal mucosal congestion and lymphadenopathy, and sometimes a harsh cough. The palpebral conjunctivae may be intensely injected or congested in the acute stage (**222**). Characteristic, small, raised, red plaques are visible near the lateral canthus. Secondary infection

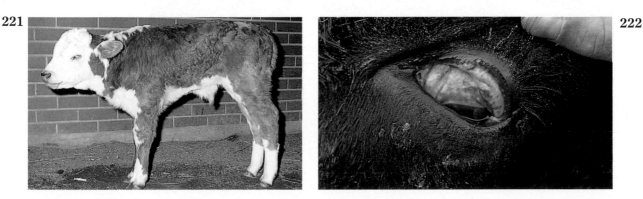

221

222

may lead to a purulent oculonasal discharge (**223**). A typical purulent IBR conjunctivitis, without blepharospasm, is shown in a Holstein cow (**224**). *Pasteurella* species are common secondary invaders. Postmortem examination (**225**) of advanced cases reveals a necrotising laryngotracheitis and areas of hyperaemia. In severe cases the nasal septum (**226**) sloughs its necrotic mucosa. Haemorrhage may follow the rupture of mucosal vessels. IBR is caused by bovine herpesvirus 1 (BHVI). Other major syndromes due to BHVI include abortion and genital tract infections. Balanoposthitis is manifested by the development of multiple, pale pustules, some of which are confluent, in the preputial mucosa. The reflection of the prepuce onto the penis is to the right (**227**). In **228**, the separated vulval lips reveal the multiple, discrete pustules of infectious pustular vulvovaginitis (IPVV). The similarity of the male and female lesions is obvious.

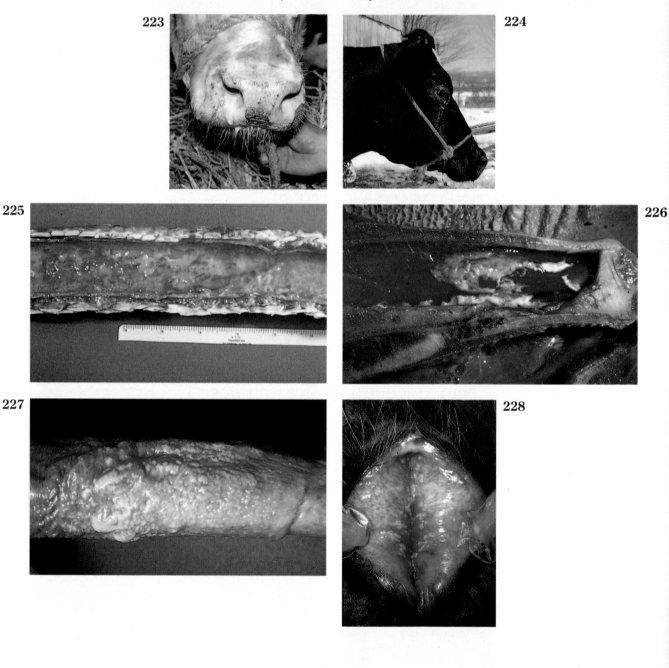

Pasteurellosis ('shipping fever', 'transit fever')

Stress, particularly that induced by transport, predisposes young cattle to pneumonic pasteurellosis, which is usually caused by *Pasteurella haemolytica*. Severe respiratory distress (**229**), with the head and neck extended, open-mouth breathing, and froth on the lips, is obvious in this standing calf, which died an hour after the photograph was taken. At postmortem examination of another calf (**230**), the apical and cardiac lobes are typically dark red, slightly swollen, firm and contain microabscesses. Such lungs may have fibrin deposits on the pleural surface. Lung changes tend to be symmetrical. A fibrinous lobar pneumonia (**231**), with red-brown consolidated areas and thickened interlobular septa, as well as bronchioles plugged with fibrinopurulent exudate, is seen on section of a well-established pasteurella pneumonia. In **232** the pneumonic areas show scattered, pale yellow abscesses. (See also *Haemophilus somnus*, **475**.)

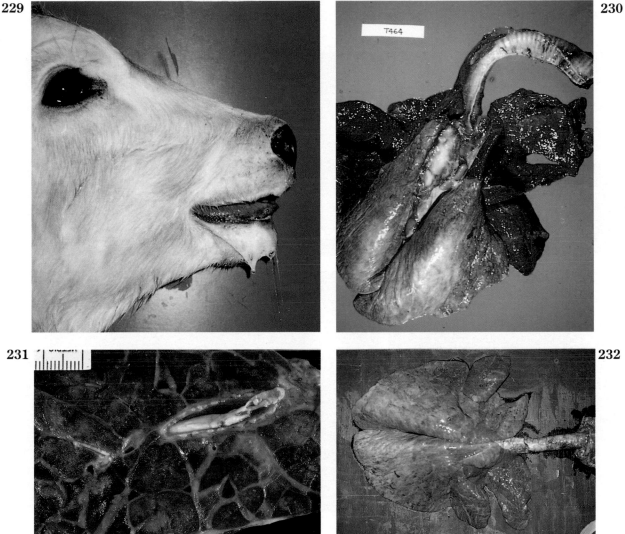

Endemic (enzootic) calf pneumonia

Endemic calf pneumonia is a broad and ill-defined entity, covering infectious pulmonary disease in young cattle that is unassociated with transport stress, but frequently related to overcrowded conditions indoors or in yards. The aetiology and epidemiology are controversial (see Introduction). The first signs are often serous ocular discharge and mild conjunctivitis (**233**). Later, a secondary infection (often *Pasteurella*) can cause a bilateral mucopurulent nasal discharge (**234**). Some calves (**235**) develop a 'sweaty' coat with damp and matted hair. Similar coat changes can also be seen in some healthy, fast-growing calves on a high-concentrate feed.

The lungs contain pink-grey or purplish areas of consolidation typically in the apical and cardiac lobes and usually (**236**) without overlying fibrin. Secondary infection can lead to pulmonary abscessation. In respiratory syncytial virus (RSV) infection all lung lobes may potentially be affected. These RSV lungs typically show areas of emphysematous bullae (A) and patchy consolidation (B), which in this calf (**237**) are in the caudal (diaphragmatic) lobes.

233
234
235
236
237

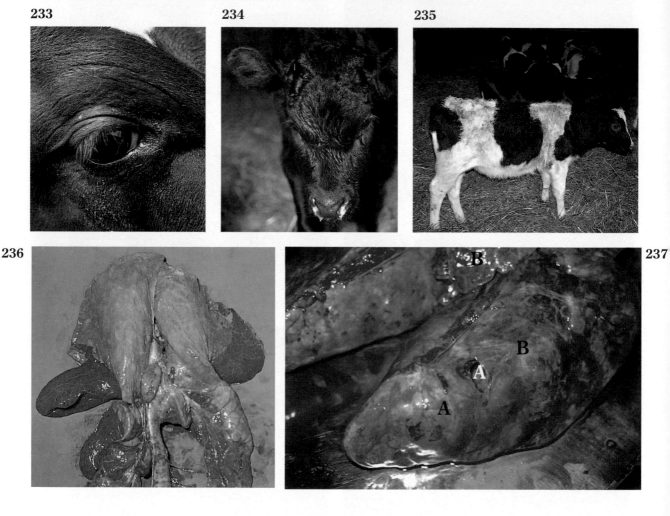

Chronic suppurative pneumonia

Chronic pneumonia is often suppurative, and many organisms can be involved. Cattle of all ages can be affected. The dull beef heifer in **238** shows typical signs of chronic pneumonia, including loss of condition, an extended tongue, head and neck, and severe dyspnoea, leading to froth on the lips. A profuse muco-purulent nasal discharge is also often seen in chronic suppurative pneumonia, together with a persistent cough. Postmortem examination (**239**) shows darkened areas of consolidation (A), emphysematous bullae (B), and abscessation (C). (See also **475**.)

238

239

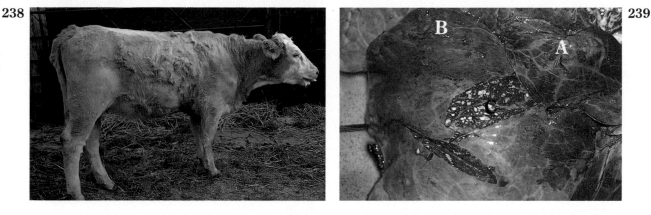

Contagious bovine pleuropneumonia

Caused by *Mycoplasma mycoides mycoides*, contagious bovine pleuropneumonia (CBPP) is a highly contagious pulmonary disease that is often accompanied by pleurisy. It continues to be rampant in many parts of Africa, India and China, and minor outbreaks occur in the Middle East. CBPP has been eradicated from North America, most of Europe (except the Iberian peninsula and parts of the Balkans), and Australia. Eradication is difficult because some infected animals become carriers and the efficacy of available vaccines is relatively poor. In most countries all outbreaks of CBPP must be notified to the central animal health authorities.

CBPP infection arises predominantly from droplet inhalation in susceptible cattle, and occasionally from ingestion of infected urine or placentae. In susceptible herds the morbidity may reach 100%, the mortality 50%, and 50% of the survivors may become carriers. The main postmortem features are a severe serofibrinous pleurisy (**240**) and fibrinonecrotic pneumonia. In **241** note the interlobular septa (A) distended by fibrinous exudate. The darker areas of lung (B) are undergoing consolidation and necrosis.

240

241

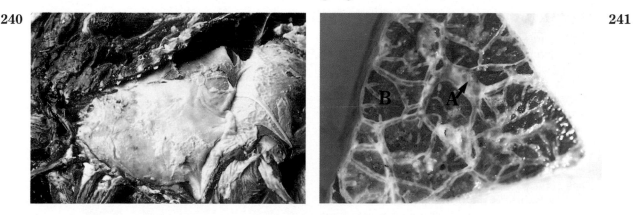

Chronic lung lesions include large sequestra (**242**) containing viable organisms, which act as an important reservoir of infection. The material can be projected as an infectious aerosol by carrier cattle which may be clinically normal. *Differential diagnosis*: acute pasteurellosis (**229–232**).

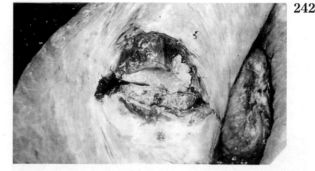

242

Tuberculosis

Bovine tuberculosis is caused by *Mycobacterium tuberculosis bovis* and is transmissible to man, usually via infected milk. Bovine organs commonly infected with tuberculosis include the alimentary tract, udder and lungs. Lung lesions have areas of yellow-orange pus that frequently become caseous. In **243** the proximity of the tuberculous lesion (A) to a bronchus could soon have made this animal capable of airborne transmission. Similar, gross, granulomatous nodules may develop beneath the intestinal mucosa (**244**). While many countries have now eradicated the disease, tuberculosis acquired from cattle remains a major human health hazard in parts of Africa, the Indian subcontinent and the Far East, where the slow, chronic nature of the infection makes early clinical diagnosis difficult.

243

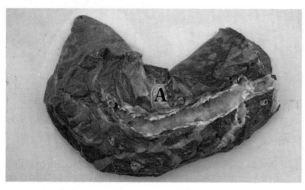

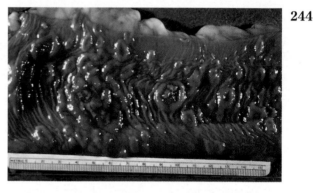

244

Lungworm infection (verminous bronchitis, 'husk')

The cattle lungworm, *Dictyocaulus viviparus*, causes bronchitis and pneumonia in young animals exposed to infective larvae during the first grazing season. The problem is primarily seen in the temperate areas of northwestern Europe. Clinical disease does not usually occur until the late summer and autumn. Early (prepatent) infection is seen as tachypnoea and partial anorexia. In later stages a persistent cough develops and the calf tends to stand with its head and neck extended (**245**), owing to bronchial irritation from the presence of the patent forms of *D. viviparus*. A characteristic, late feature is the development of a chronic, nonsuppurative, eosinophilic granulomatous pneumonia, primarily in the caudal lobes of the lung.

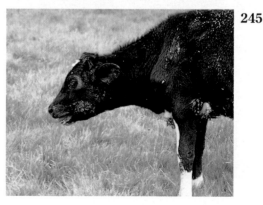

245

Considerable weight loss results, and in those cases that recover, there this reduced weight again. Post-mortem examination of a severe case (**246**) shows huge numbers of maturing larvae in the bronchi and bronchioles. Reinfection can occur in adult cattle (usually in dairy cows in the autumn) in the form of an extensive eosinophilic bronchitis. Larvae may be demonstrated in the faeces or oronasal mucus of advanced cases. An oral vaccine of irradiated larvae is available.

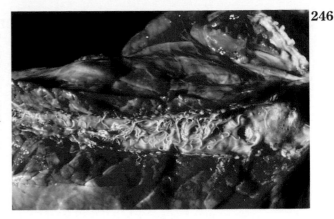

246

Atypical interstitial pneumonia (bovine pulmonary emphysema, enzootic bovine adenomatosis, 'fog fever', 'panters')

247

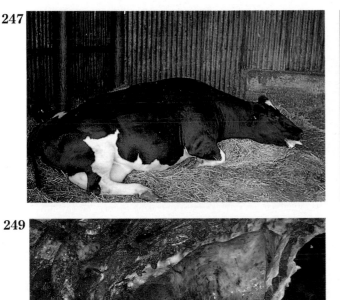

248

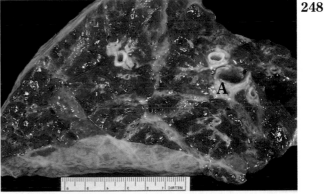

249

Atypical interstitial pneumonia or acute respiratory distress syndrome occurs predominantly in adult beef cattle, and, to a lesser extent, in dairy cattle. It typically follows a change from bare grazing onto lush pastures in the autumn. Severe respiratory distress (**247**) is seen, with drooling of saliva, and open-mouth breathing. The lungs of acute cases (**248**) are heavy and have extensive areas of oedema and emphysema (A), some of which may form large bullae (**248 & 249**). The amino acid, D,L-tryptophan, the levels of which are high in lush autumn pastures, is thought to be a significant cause of this type of pneumonia, the actual toxic agent being a metabolite of D,L-tryptophan, 3-methylindole, that is produced in the rumen. Some cases have an uncertain aetiology.

Aspiration pneumonia (inhalation pneumonia)

The right thoracic wall has been removed from a Holstein cow to show the effects of accidental aspiration of mineral oil (liquid paraffin) about 60 hours previously (**250**). The entire surface of the visible pleura covering the lungs appears greasy as a result of oil leakage through ruptured bullae. Severe interlobular oedema and emphysema are evident. Affected lobes may also reveal congestion, and early necrosis. Foreign body aspiration (drenches, rumen fluid) is frequently fatal within 48–72 hours.

250

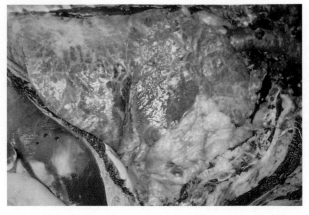

Pulmonary thromboembolism (caudal vena caval thrombosis)

251

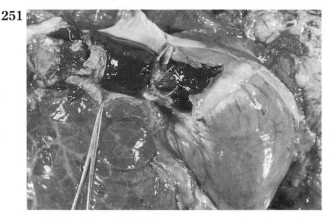

252

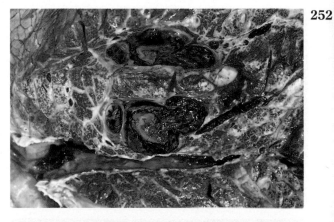

253

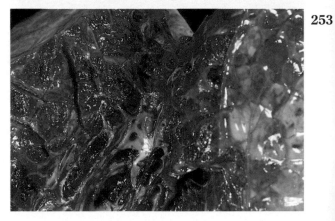

The complex aetiology of the dramatic syndrome, pulmonary thromboembolism, (PTE-CVC) starts with hepatic abscessation, often from rumenitis, leading to a localised caudal vena caval thrombosis (**251**). The haemostat holds the wall of the CVC. Bacteraemia may cause seeding of the lungs with septic emboli, some of which may be massive (**252**). Emphysema, thrombosis and oedematous changes are seen in the lungs of the four-year-old Hereford bull in **253**. Pulmonary arterial lesions can cause thromboembolism, aneurysm formation and severe intrabronchial haemorrhage, haemoptysis, anaemia, and melaena from swallowed blood.

In a fatal haemoptysis resulting from PTE-CVC (254), frothy arterial blood is seen on the bedding and walls of a stall. Septic emboli may spread to other organs, and renal infarction (255) is common. The dark areas (A) in the renal cortex are recent infarcts; the paler areas (B) are older. PTE-CVC affects animals of all ages.

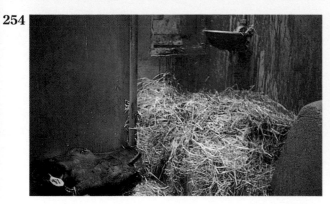

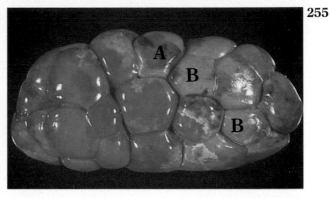

Brisket disease (altitude sickness)

Brisket disease results from congestive cardiac failure at high altitudes (usually above 2,500 metres), where impairment of the circulatory or respiratory system overcomes the cardiac reserve capacity and causes chronic physiological hypoxia. The Hereford heifer (256) from Colorado, USA, shows pronounced submandibular and presternal oedema, depression and dehydration.

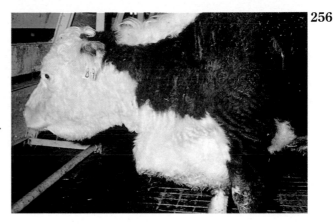

6 Cardiovascular disorders

Introduction

This chapter is short not because cardiovascular disorders are uncommon, but because many conditions are illustrated in other chapters. Three basic cardiac syndromes encompass most disorders: the first is congestive cardiac failure, which may result from valvular disease (**259–262**), myocardial or pericardial disease (**263–265**), hypertension, or congenital defects which produce shunts (**23–25**). Secondly, and less commonly, an acute heart failure can result from tachyarrhythmia caused by a nutritional deficiency myopathy (e.g., copper or selenium), electrocution or a lightning strike (classified under nervous disorders,

487–490), or bradycardia due to plant poisoning by *Solanum, Trisetum* and *Lantana* species, all of which can induce myocardial changes (**710–713**). Thirdly, peripheral circulatory failure can result from peripheral vasodilatation and a reduced circulating blood volume as in septic shock (e.g., acute gangrenous mastitis and acute metritis), or endotoxic shock from a peracute coliform mastitis (**583–588**). Peripheral circulatory failure can also be due to haematogenic failure (as a result of severe haemorrhage, see **254**), or as a consequence of neonatal calf diarrhoea (**40–48**).

Congestive cardiac failure

In heart failure the venous return may be impaired as a result of the right side of the heart failing to pump blood to the lungs. Jugular venous distension may then be marked (jugular cording), as seen in the Friesian cow in **257**. Poor venous return resulted in the development of a dependent oedema, particularly

submandibular, presternal (**258**) and later, ventral abdominal. The cow was dull, pyrexic and developed a chronic cough as a result of passive venous congestion. Ventral oedema due to circulatory failure should be distinguished from a transient peripartum oedema which is normal in dairy cows (see **626**).

257

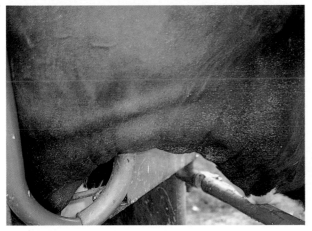

258

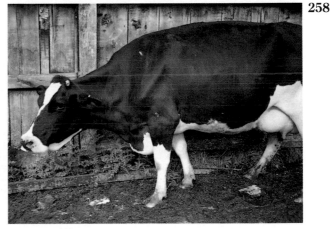

Vegetative or nodular endocarditis

Another cause of congestive cardiac failure, bovine endocarditis may involve septicaemia resulting from a remote focus, such as an infected joint or the umbilicus. Alternatively, the lesion may develop slowly in adult cattle, which remain asymptomatic, and manifest no evidence of bacterial infection (endocardiosis). This section illustrates bacterial endocarditis. The Guernsey cow in **259** developed a massive abscess involving the left subcutaneous abdominal vein (milk vein), which caused severe valvular endocarditis and death. Some cases that occur in young calves (**260**)

may have prominent valvular nodules from which *Pasteurella haemolytica* and alpha-haemolytic streptococci can be isolated, suggesting that the original infection involved the respiratory tract. Some lesions in vegetative endocarditis are fleshy red, indicative of recent deposition and growth, generally along the right atrioventricular valve cusps and leaflets (**261**). Other cases appear yellowish-red and may almost obliterate the leaflets, as in the six-year-old Holstein cow (**262**), from which streptococci were isolated.

259

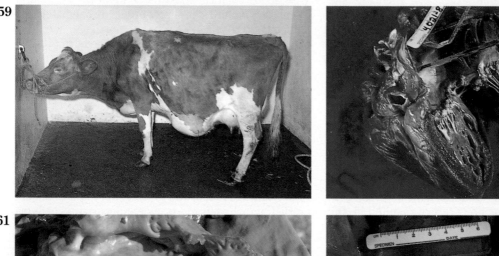

260

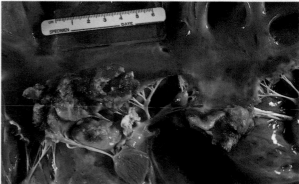

261

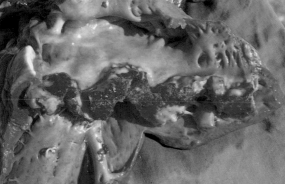

262

Septic pericarditis and myocarditis

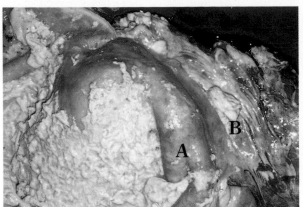

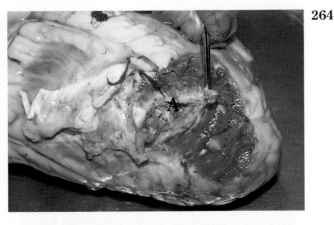

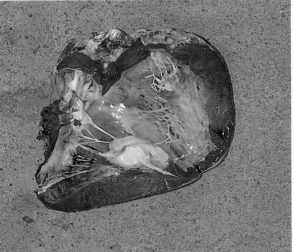

Septic pericarditis is usually a sequel to penetration of the pericardial sac by a wire that has migrated from the reticulum through the diaphragm. Congestive cardiac failure is the result. In the Charolais bull in **263** a massive volume of yellow pus ('scrambled egg' appearance) occupies the pericardial sac. The surface (A) below the pus is the thickened, partly fibrosed epicardium. The thickness of the pericardial wall can be judged from the depth of the sternum (B). Heart failure may result from migration of the foreign body (wire, A) into the myocardium itself (**264**). Ventral oedema is often a sequel to septic pericarditis caused by traumatic reticulitis. The absence of a septic track from the reticulum through the diaphragm to the pericardium and heart, indicates that fatal myocardial abscessation can sometimes arise through haematogenous infection. In this cow (**265**), in which the original septic focus was a septic pedal arthritis, the abscess involves the papillary muscles and myocardium.

7 Locomotor disorders

Lower limb and digit
Introduction

In dairy cattle, approximately 80% of all lameness originates in the foot, particularly in the hind feet. Lameness is a major cause of economic loss, as affected animals lose weight rapidly, yields fall and, in protracted cases, fertility is affected. There is also increased culling, and considerable sums of money are spent on treatment and preventive hoof trimming. Although accurate figures are not available, lameness in beef cattle has a lower incidence and less economic importance. There are many aetiological factors involved, including excessive standing, especially on hard, unyielding surfaces, feet kept continually wet in corrosive slurry, and high concentrate/low fibre feeding systems which can precipitate acidosis and subsequent laminitis. The consequences of laminitis are an abnormal stance and hoof wear, softening of the sole horn and a weakening and widening of the white line, all of which predispose to digital lameness.

This chapter illustrates the common foot lesions in cattle, namely white line abscess, foreign body penetration of the sole, sole ulcer, interdigital necrobacillosis, interdigital skin hyperplasia and digital dermatitis. Complications of these primary conditions may produce deeper digital infections, involving the navicular bursa and, eventually, the pedal (distal interphalangeal) joint. Flexor tendon rupture or coronary band abscessation may result. The final section deals with vertical and horizontal claw fissures (sandcracks), claw overgrowth and laminitis. Digital lesions due to systemic disease, e.g., foot-and-mouth (**632** & **633**) are described in the relevant chapters.

Disorders of the sole (bearing surface) and axial wall

White line impaction

The white line is the junction between the sole horn and the hoof wall. It is a point of weakness in the hoof, and the most common site for the entry of dirt and infection. **266** illustrates white line impaction: on the abaxial aspect of the right claw the white line has been grossly expanded by stones and mixed, black detritus. Infection may eventually reach the laminae (also known as the pododerm or corium), leading to lameness. The sole horn has a yellow waxy appearance and is of poor quality. Slight sole haemorrhage can be seen on the left claw, and the heels show horn erosion (black areas). The toes have been clipped in the course of foot-trimming.

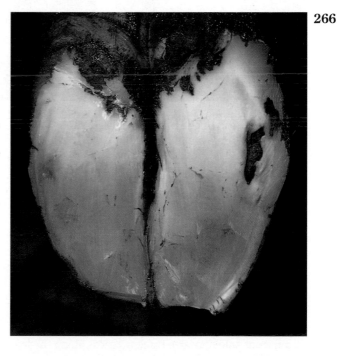

266

False sole

In this oblique view, removal of the impacted white line from the animal in **266** revealed an area of under-run sole (at the point of the hypodermic needle), with underlying new horn (**267**). The superficial layer of separated horn is often called a false sole. This cow was not lame.

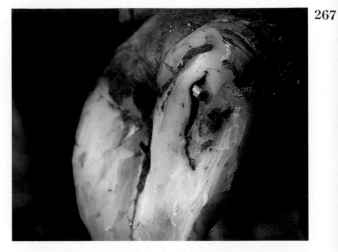

White line abscess

268

269

270

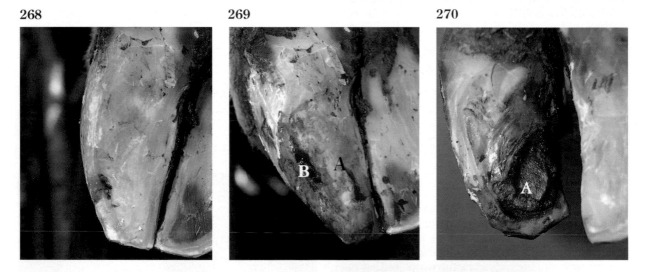

On the left claw (**268**) light greyish pus is exuding from the point of entry of infection at the white line near the toe. Pus has tracked under the sole horn, leading to separation of the horn from the laminae. Lameness was pronounced. In **269** the underrun sole has been removed to expose new sole horn, developing as a layer of creamy-white tissue (A) in the centre of the sole and against the edge of the trimmed horn. The haemorrhagic area (B) at the white line is the original point of entry of infection. Progressively deeper penetration of infection occurs in untreated cases. In **270**, another sole view, the corium has been eroded to expose the tip of the pedal bone (A). This resulted in severe lameness, although the cow eventually made a full recovery. Infection in the white line or adjacent sole may also track upwards along the laminae of the hoof wall to discharge at the coronary band (**271**). (Compare with **268**, where infection underruns

271

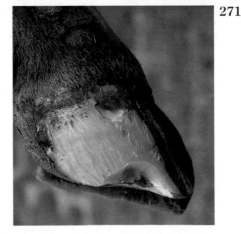

the sole horn.) In **272**, the infected track, the brown necrotic line (A), has been exposed to provide drainage. A wooden block has been glued onto the sound claw, to rest the affected digit. Although this cow walked soundly within three weeks, more than 12 months elapsed before sufficient horn had grown down from the coronet to repair the damaged hoof. An increased incidence of white line separation and abscess formation may occur when cattle walk on rough surfaces or tracks where there are small, sharp flints, or as a consequence of softening of the hoof.

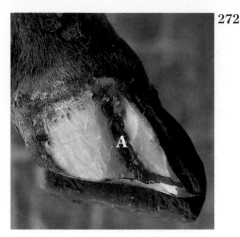
272

Foreign body penetration of the sole

273

274

275

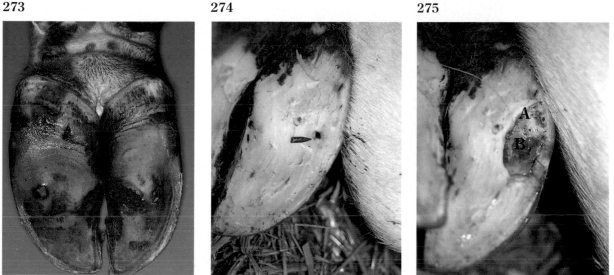

In **273** a stone is firmly impacted in the sole, towards the heel. Note the slight swelling of the heel. Unless the stone penetrates the sole horn, leading to infection and underrun laminae, lameness is relatively mild. Stones and nails are the most common foreign bodies. The dark marks on other areas of the soles of both claws are indicative of old bruises. In **274** a portion of nail has penetrated the sole horn on the axial aspect of the white line, carrying infection into the laminae. In **275** superficial horn has been removed to provide drainage and to expose the new sole (A) developing beneath. In the centre (B) is the sensitive matrix. Sole puncture at the toe can cause osteomyelitis of the distal phalanx or pedal bone (**276**). Note the haemorrhagic and necrotic areas beneath the wall (A) and solar separation (B). (See also **270**.)

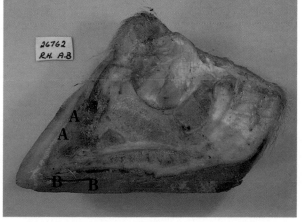
276

Axial wall penetration

Foreign body penetration of the axial wall in the heifer in **277** resulted in a localised septic laminitis (A), with secondary interdigital swelling and necrosis. The wall is thinnest at this point, i.e., the junction of the heel, sole and axial wall horn.

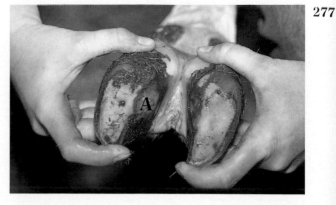

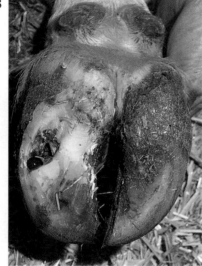

278

Sole abscess

Note the large sole cavity (**278**), which was originally filled with dark grey pus, and the new horn (A) forming on the underlying laminae. The size of the cavity and the extent of new horn formation indicate a more chronic case than that in **268**. The enlarged heel bulb suggests secondary involvement. Infection originally penetrated through the white line.

Abscess at the coronary band

Infection originating at the white line has passed proximally under the hoof wall to the coronet in **279**, where it has penetrated the deeper tissues of the collateral digital ligaments to produce a septic cellulitis. As well as highlighting the overgrowth of the sole horn, this chronic lesion shows that the horn wall is detached from the coronet beneath the abscess. The affected toe has deviated dorsally, leading to relative overgrowth from lack of wear.

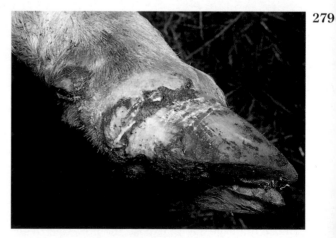

Abscess at heel

Note the marked unilateral enlargement of the left heel in **280**, with inflammation tracking up towards the fetlock and causing distortion of the claw. The navicular bursa and pedal joint are also infected, pro-ducing a septic pedal arthritis. Gross pedal enlargement in **281** has led to lifting of sole and heel horn, especially towards the interdigital space.

280
281

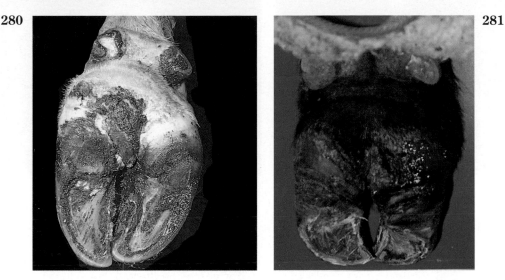

Deep sepsis

Septic pedal arthritis (distal interphalangeal sepsis)

Pedal arthritis typically results from a neglected white line abscess, sole ulcer or interdigital infection. The Hereford cow in **282** had been lame for eight weeks. The affected (lateral) left claw is grossly enlarged and inflamed, there is swelling of the coronet and separa-tion of horn at the coronary band (A), and granulation tissue protrudes into the interdigital space at the point where pus discharges from the infected joint. Despite a less severe degree of swelling in the more chronic case in **283**, the hoof on the affected lateral (right) claw is being evulsed by pressure and necrosis from a septic coronitis.

282
283

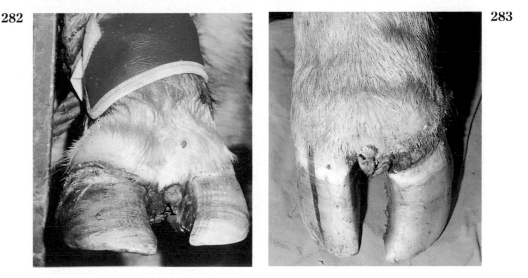

In a longitudinal section of a claw (**284**), purulent infection can be seen in the digital cushion (A) adjacent to the navicular bone, the deep digital flexor tendon (B) and the pedal joint (C). In **285**, which is a sagittal section following digital amputation, necrosis in the navicular bone has extended to cause severe sepsis in the distal joint (A). Infection at the coronary band (B) has produced swelling above the coronet.

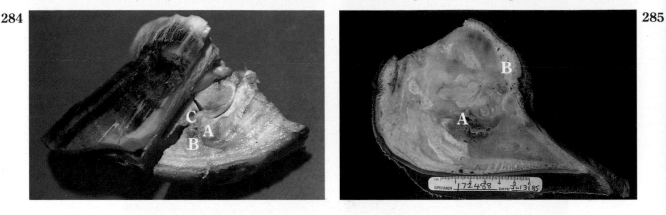

Rupture of the deep flexor tendon

Complications from severe white line abscessation, a sole ulcer, or, as in **286**, a heel abscess, can lead to infection and the subsequent rupture of the deep flexor tendon. The coronary band is severely distorted, the heel is swollen and the toe deviates upwards (plantigrade), leading to continual overgrowth and lack of wear of the affected claw. A longitudinal section of a septic digit (**287**) reveals the site of the ulcer that perforated the sole horn (A), and the point of rupture of the deep flexor tendon (B).

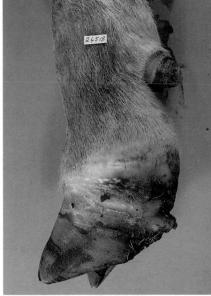

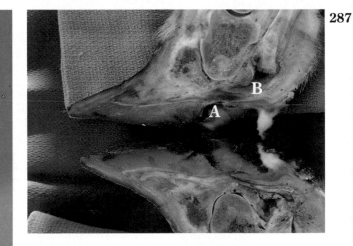

Sole ulceration

The digit in **288** (a plantar view) has a wedge of sole horn (A) growing from the axial aspect of the right (lateral) claw towards the left claw. This wedge increasingly becomes a major weight-bearing surface and transmits excess weight to the sole laminae, causing haemorrhage, bruising and, eventually, pressure necrosis. Note also the heel erosion (B). **289** shows that when such a sole wedge is pared away, a discrete area of sole haemorrhage is exposed in the right (lateral) claw. Note the reddening of the white line in the same claw, indicative of laminitis, and also that both claws are badly overgrown. Further paring and removal of the haemorrhagic horn (**290**) reveal underrun horn and necrosis characteristic of a sole

ulcer. The axial wedge of sole overgrowth is less pronounced in the left (lateral) claw in **291**, although pressure on this wedge produced pain and a bloody discharge into the interdigital space. Removal of the wedge exposes a typical sole ulcer (**292**), with a large, protruding mass of granulation tissue. The longitudinal section of another case (**293**) illustrates a mild, chronic ulcer in its characteristic site at the sole–heel junction. The sole horn has been perforated (A) and inflammatory changes have tracked up towards the insertion of the deep flexor tendon. The heel horn is slightly underrun (B) and there is laminitic haemorrhage at the toe (C). Neglected ulcers may

288

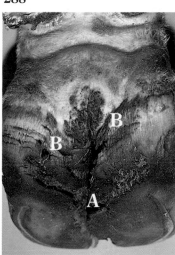

289

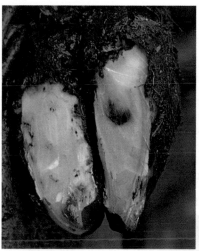

290

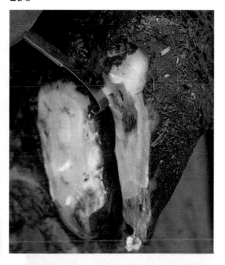

291

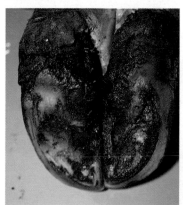

292

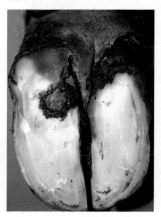

293

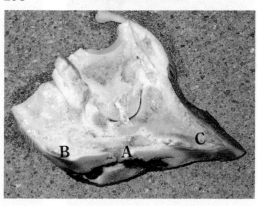

penetrate deeper structures: **294** shows heel enlargement, and a purulent exudate from an infected navicular bursa discharging through the original ulcer site. A wooden block has been applied to the sound claw. Flexor tendon rupture (**287**) may result from complicated cases. Ulcers are typically found on the lateral claws of hind feet and, less frequently, on the medial claws of front feet. Often the lateral digits of both hind feet are involved. More extensive damage to the laminae means that they heal more slowly than a white line abscess or an underrun sole (**269**). Herd outbreaks may be seen following ruminal acidosis (excess concentrate/inadequate dietary fibre), or as a consequence of prolonged standing on a hard surface, for example, following a change from loose yards to cubicle (free-stall) housing. Poor cubicle design and inadequate bedding, leading to reduced use, are also important.

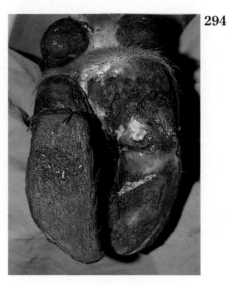

294

Disorders of the interdigital space and heels

Interdigital necrobacillosis (phlegmona interdigitalis, 'foul', 'footrot')

A common cause of lameness, interdigital necrobacillosis is an infection of the interdigital skin associated with *Fusobacterium necrophorum* and other bacteria. Infection starts in the dermis. Early cases show a symmetrical, bilateral, hyperaemic swelling of the heel bulbs (**295**) that sometimes extends to the accessory digits. At this stage, the interdigital skin is swollen but intact, and the claws appear to be pushed apart when the animal stands (**296**). After 24–48 hours the interdigital skin splits (**297**) (some sloughed epidermis has been removed), and in later cases,

295

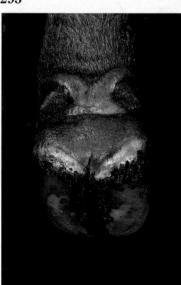

296

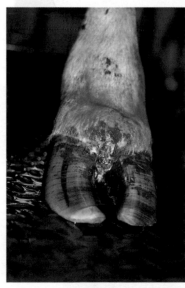

297

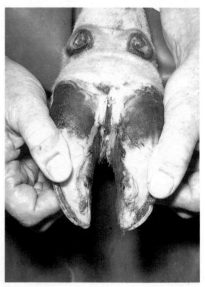

the dermis is exposed (**298**). There may be a foul-smelling, caseous exudate, as seen in **296**. **299** is a dorsal view of a neglected case after cleansing, with sloughed, necrotic debris in the interdigital space. The depth of the necrotic process has caused proliferation of granulation tissue. Early separation of the axial wall of the left claw (A) and swelling of the coronet suggest the presence of early inflammatory changes in the pedal joint. The horizontal groove (B) distal to the coronary band indicates that the problem has existed for about one month. *Differential diagnosis*: interdigital dermatitis (**308**).

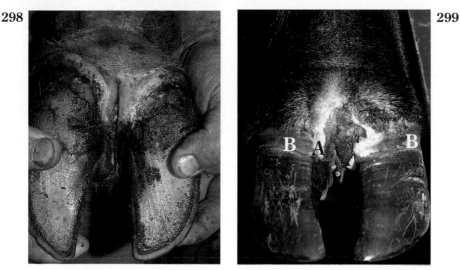

Interdigital skin hyperplasia (fibroma, 'corn')

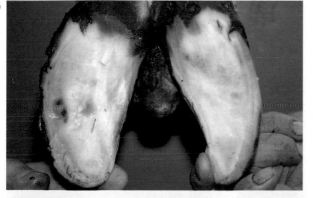

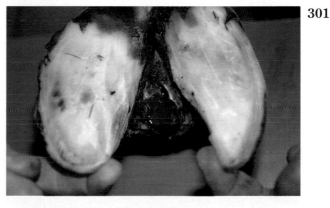

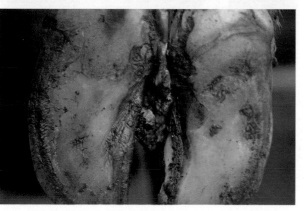

Hyperplasia in the interdigital space develops from skin folds adjacent to the axial hoof wall, as shown in **300**. Note the sole haemorrhage due to bruising of the left claw. This type of lesion, which is often symmetrical, is a particular problem in mature beef bulls. Cows are also affected. The condition may be inherited. Surgical removal exposes the dermis (**301**) and demonstrates the extent to which the claws are forced apart by the hyperplasia. Lameness is produced either when the claws pinch the interdigital skin during walking, or following secondary (necrobacillary) infection in areas of pressure necrosis (**302**). Note the superficial but severe slough of necrotic material.

In a few cases, hyperplasia is restricted more to the dorsal interdigital space (**303**), when lameness is less likely. *Differential diagnosis*: interdigital necrobacillosis (**295**).

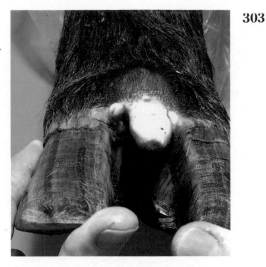

303

Digital dermatitis

Digital dermatitis is a superficial epidermitis that is associated with cows standing in slurry. It may involve *Bacteroides* species. The lesion is typically seen on the skin above the heel bulbs, proximal to the interdigital space. On initial inspection, early cases (**304**) show hairs (A) that are erect and matted with a serous exudate. Cleaning superficial debris (**305**) reveals a circular area of epidermitis, 1–2 cm in diameter. Affected animals are acutely lame, even though dermal tissues are not significantly involved (compare interdigital

304

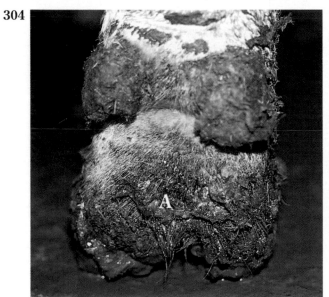

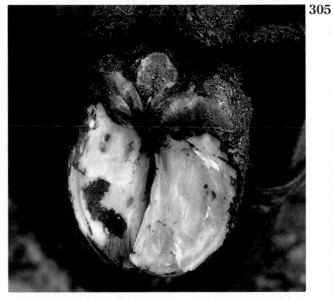

305

necrobacillosis, **295**). In advanced lesions (**306**) the heel horn becomes eroded and underrun, with an extensive raw area of epidermitis extending up towards the accessory digits. Such advanced lesions may require surgical correction. Although the majority of cases occur at the plantar aspect, ulcerating dorsal lesions, as seen in **307**, are not uncommon. Such lesions, involving perioplic horn of the coronary band, may produce a more protracted lameness. Formalin and antibiotic footbaths have been introduced in herd outbreaks with varying success, but topical treatment is surprisingly effective. *Differential diagnosis*: necrobacillosis (**295**), interdigital dermatitis (**308**), mud fever (**310**), and heel erosion or slurry heel (**311**).

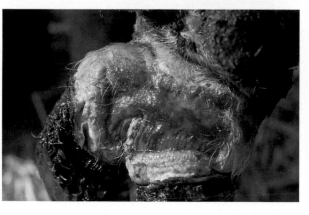

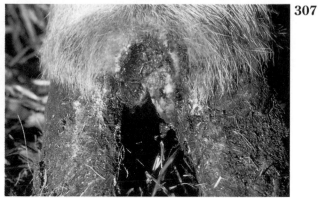

Interdigital dermatitis

Interdigital dermatitis is a superficial, moist inflammation of the interdigital epidermis (**308**) that does not involve the deeper tissues, and hence differs from necrobacillosis (**295**). *Bacteroides nodosus* has occasionally been recovered from lesions. Despite the superficial nature of the lesion, lameness is often pronounced. Many consider that this lesion is related to digital dermatitis.

Papillomata in the interdigital space

In **309** the multiple, fine papillomata protruding from the skin between the bulbs of the heels are a result of chronic skin irritation. A digital dermatitis lesion has been suggested as a predisposing factor.

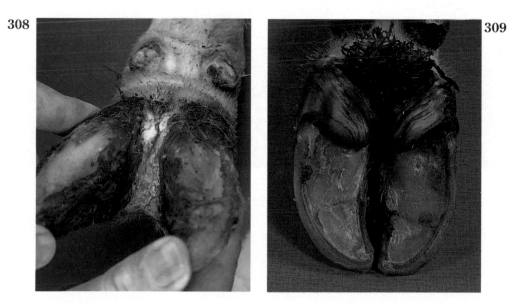

'Mud fever'

Mud fever occurs following exposure to cold, wet, muddy conditions and may involve secondary *Dermatophilus* infection (see **96**). In **310** the skin is thickened with a dry eczema and there is hair loss from the heel bulbs, extending upwards to the fetlock. The superficial haemorrhage resulted from cleaning. Lameness is pronounced and all four limbs may be affected. *Differential diagnosis*: digital dermatitis (**304**).

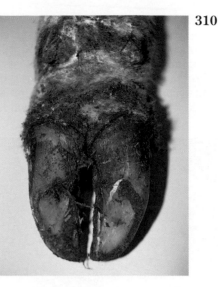

310

Heel erosion ('slurry heel')

The heel is an important weight-bearing surface. Its intact structure has been demonstrated in preceding illustrations, e.g., **298**. Erosion is commonly seen in housed dairy cows that stand in slurry. In **311** the original smooth horn has been eroded, producing a deep fissure in the left heel. In a severe case involving both heels (**312**), erosion of the right (lateral) heel horn has led to the appearance of granulation tissue from the sole. Loss of the heel horn destabilises the hoof, alters weight-bearing, increases concussion, and may predispose to sole ulcers. Slurry heel may be related to digital and interdigital dermatitis. *Bacteroides nodosus* has occasionally been isolated from both lesions. **313** illustrates erosion of both heels, with an area of digital dermatitis (A) at the heel–horn junction on the right claw.

311

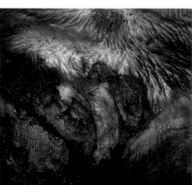

312

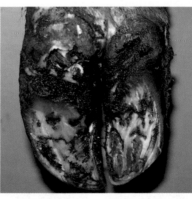

313

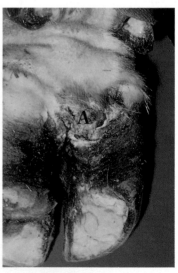

Interdigital foreign body

In **314** a stone is impacted in the interdigital space, ulcerating the axial skin of the left claw. Small pieces of twig, especially thorns, can lie longitudinally in the cleft, damaging the interdigital skin and leading to secondary necrobacillosis.

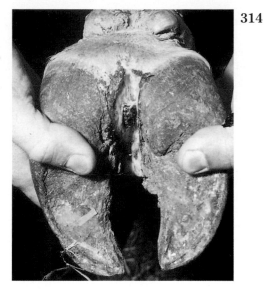

314

Disorders of the hoof wall

Vertical fissure (vertical sandcrack)

Sandcracks occur as a result of damage to the superficial periople, for example, following hot, dry weather, or damage to the coronary band. Both claws of the overgrown left forefoot in **315** are affected, although the major fissure appears only on the medial claw. Note its irregular course and its origin at the coronary band (A). Note also the section (B), which is slightly loose due to an oblique crack at (C). In **316** only the right claw is affected. Despite being limited to the distal third of the claw, the fissure is much deeper and the toe is broken off. An extensive, wide, vertical horn crack is shown, in which the laminae are very liable to become exposed, resulting in severe lameness, even though little pus may be present. In advanced cases (**317**), granulation tissue with blood may protrude from the fissure.

315   **316**   **317**

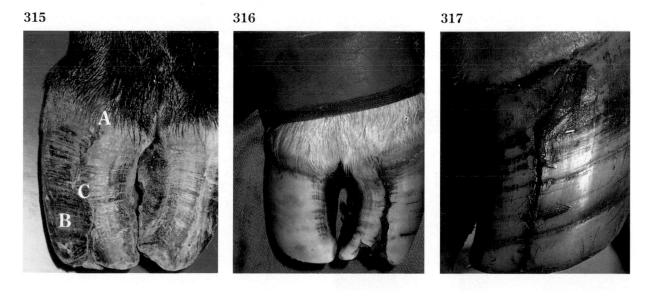

Horizontal fissure (horizontal sandcrack)

In **318** both claws are affected: the hand-held, cracked, medial hoof wall resulted from a temporary cessation of horn formation four months previously, due to an abrupt dietary change. The 'thimble' of loose horn will eventually grow out at the toe. Lameness results from the pressure of the hinged portion of horn on the underlying laminae, or from exposure of the sensitive laminae when the thimble becomes detached (broken toe). In **318** a smaller fissure of the lateral claw has been partially trimmed off, without exposing sensitive laminae, to reduce the amount of movement of the thimble. With some cows, both claws of all four feet may be affected as a result of a severe systemic insult, for example following acute mastitis or acute metritis.

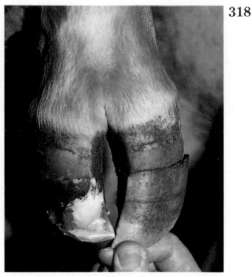

318

Corkscrew claw

319

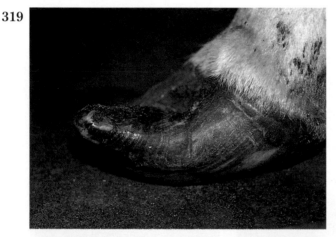

320

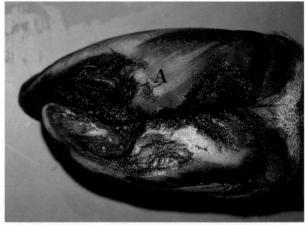

321

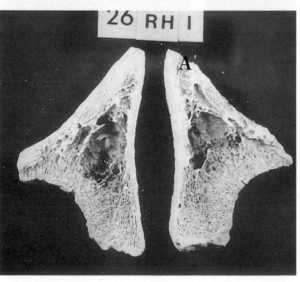

The lateral claw of the front or the hind feet can be affected by this partially heritable growth defect. The overgrown lateral toe in **319** deviates upwards, and in the same digit, the abaxial wall curls under the sole (**320**), inevitably altering the weight-bearing surfaces. The axial sole overgrowth (**320, A**) consequently becomes a major weight-bearing surface and lameness can result from sole ulcers and/or pedal bone compression (see also **291 & 323**). In the pedal bone specimen in **321**, osteolysis secondary to corkscrew claw compression is seen near the toe, at A. The left pedal bone and the cavitation are normal. **320** also shows early bilateral heel erosion (see also **312**), and cavitation of the sole of the medial claw due to impaction by debris.

Scissor claw

322

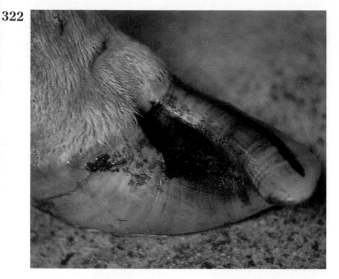

Scissor claw differs from corkscrew claw in that one toe grows across the other, there is less wall involvement, and rotation along a longitudinal axis is absent. In **322** the wall of the left claw curls slightly axially at the point of contact with the ground, and may form a false sole. Slight mechanical lameness can result from the pressure of one toe on top of the other during walking.

Sole overgrowth

323

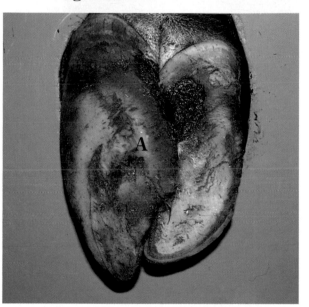

Probably the result of a chronic laminitis, the lateral (left) claw in **323** is much larger than the medial claw, and the outer wall is overgrown, curling axially towards the sole. A wedge of sole horn (A) is growing across towards the medial claw. This wedge predisposes the animal to sole bruising and/or sole ulcers (see also **288**, **291**, **303** & **320**). The black areas on the heels are early heel erosions (**312**).

Fracture of distal phalanx

Occurring primarily in the front feet, distal phalangeal fracture is usually traumatic, although it may be pathologically associated with fluorosis (**727**) or osteomyelitis. The medial claw is often involved, forcing the animal to adopt a cross-legged stance, and hence transferring weight to the lateral claw (**324**). The fracture line (A) in **325** runs vertically from the distal interphalangeal joint, and the two fragments of pedal bone are separated.

This type of fracture leads to a sudden onset of severe lameness, often with no initial visible signs of heat or swelling. Later, the affected claw may be palpably hotter, but in the early stages, diagnosis without radiography is difficult. The fracture is almost always intra-articular, unless it results from digital osteomyelitis. *Differential diagnosis*: foreign body perforation of the interdigital space or the sole.

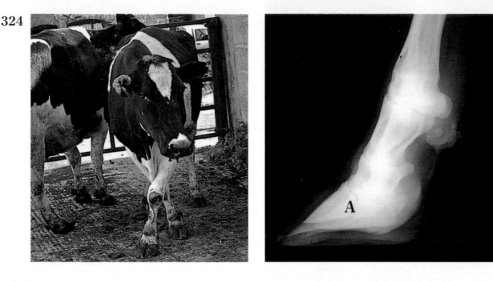

324

325

Laminitis

Acute laminitis

The Friesian cow in **326** has a typical acute laminitic stance: the front legs are abducted, the hind legs are placed forward under the abdomen, the back is arched, the neck is extended, and the tail is slightly raised. Hoof changes following laminitis are shown in **327**. Haemorrhage can be seen over the heel bulb and along the white line. Note the black debris impacted into the widened white line towards the heel, which could result in white line infection (**268**). Intense congestion of laminar blood vessels under the wall of the hoof,

leading to downward (ventral) rotation of the anterior tip of the pedal bone, is the most probable cause of the blood clot in the sole horn towards A. The heifer had calved two months previously and the laminitis was probably the result of a change from a fibrous to a high concentrate diet (producing acidosis), combined with excessive standing on concrete. The condition is frequently seen when heifers that have been reared in yards or on pasture are introduced postpartum into cubicles for the first time.

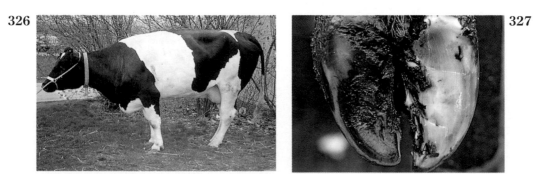

326

327

The gross widening and haemorrhage of the white line in the three-year-old Simmental bull (**328**) was the result of excessive exercise in a cubicle-housed dairy herd over several months, at the beginning of which acute laminitis developed. These changes caused softening of the white line, permitted penetration of dirt, and resulted in acute lameness due to the underrun sole. (Compare white line abscess, **268–272**.)

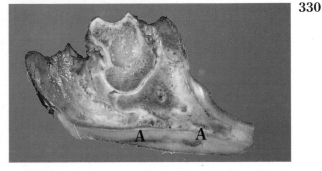

Chronic laminitis

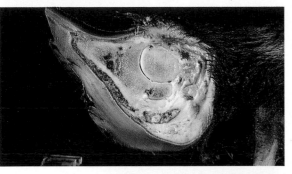

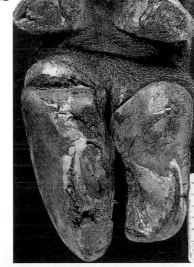

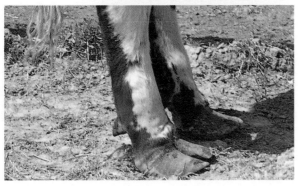

In this longitudinal section (**329**) through the foot of a six-year-old Shorthorn bull with early chronic laminitis, the sole laminae are thickened and haemorrhagic, and pink striations indicate that there is blood in the sole horn, particularly at the toe. The pedal bone is deviated downwards, away from the overlying hoof wall. At a later stage (**330**), the line of haemorrhage (A) in the sole horn beneath the pedal bone is easily recognisable. The laminitic insult responsible for this line would have occurred about five weeks previously. Note the thickening and the dorsal deviation of the toe. These changes lead to growth irregularities of the type seen in **331** & **332**. In **331** the wall of the outer claw (left) is curling axially. A deep heel fissure and an obvious false sole are developing. The medial claw (right) has an expanded white line. Both front claws in **332** are elongated and the heels are sunken. The toe angle is small, there are prominent horizontal lines, and the periople at the coronary band is flaky.

Upper limb and spine

Introduction

The illustrations in this section have been grouped primarily by affected area and type of damage. The 'downer cow' syndrome is followed by spinal conditions, and trauma affecting joints and long bones (fractures). Paralyses, excluding those illustrated in the downer cow section, form another small group. Infectious causes are illustrated in the septic arthritides section. A miscellaneous group includes vitamin and mineral deficiencies and metabolic disorders that can result in lameness.

Downer cow

Metabolic disease, and specifically a nonresponsive milk fever or hypocalcaemia (see **455** & **456**), is the major cause of the downer cow syndrome. Such cows fail to rise after treatment for hypocalcaemia. The reason often remains unknown. Lying on hard concrete or on the edge of the gutter in a standing or cubicle for as little as six hours has been shown to produce permanent nerve damage in the hind leg. Struggling may cause dislocation of the hip joint, muscle rupture, a femoral fracture or other traumatic incidents that prevent the animal from rising, despite being normocalcaemic. Other more insidious conditions, such as metritis, mastitis and toxicities, can also cause a cow or a bull to become a downer. Blood changes include a rapid elevation of muscle enzymes, such as serum glutamic-oxaloacetic transaminase (SGOT) and creatine phosphokinase (CPK), as a result of ischaemic muscle necrosis.

Management of the downer cow is very important. Good nursing on soft bedding is the prime requirement. The animal should be turned from one side to the other, several times daily. Loss of appetite and signs of dullness and toxicity suggest a poor prognosis, but some alert downers have been known to rise spontaneously after several weeks. Hip clamps, slings and inflatable bags have a role in temporarily elevating the hindquarters.

Downer cow: spinal or pelvic damage

Suddenly, after dystocia, the mature Simmental female in **333** adopted this 'dog-sitting' position, which is suggestive of lumbar or pelvic canal trauma. The posterior paresis resolved after three weeks, and the cow recovered completely. Occasionally, this position is habitual as a result of spondylarthrosis. Progress-ively severe posterior paresis with 'knuckling' of the hind fetlocks (**334**) developed in this mature Holstein as a result of vertebral lymphoma. Necropsy of a similar case (**335**) shows a transverse

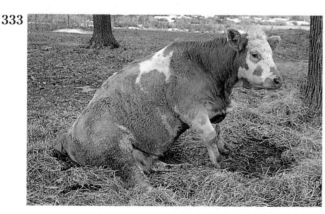

333

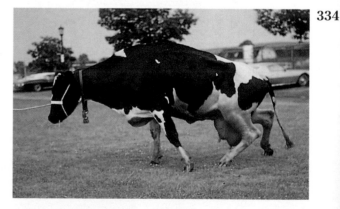

334

section of the caudal lumbar vertebral area with yellow-brown lymphomatous tissue (A) and normal, white, epidural fat within the spinal canal. The lymphoma caused marked compression of the spinal nerves, including the sciatic supply. The Friesian cow in **336** had lumbar spondylosis and stood and walked only with great difficulty. Body condition is poor and the thoracolumbar spine is convex and prominent owing to muscle atrophy. The position of the hind legs relieves pain on spinal nerves. A lateral radiograph of a similar case (**337**) shows degenerative arthropathy of the lumbar region, with ventral osteophyte proliferation (A).Progressive ankylosis brings a risk of fracture of the newly deposited bone of the spinal body, leading to the downer syndrome.

335

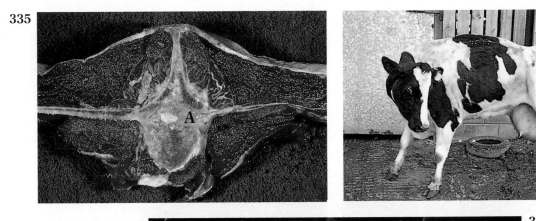

336

337

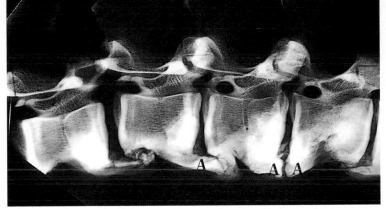

Downer cow: dislocated hip

Hip dislocation as a cause of a 'downer cow' is usually related to ventral and caudal dislocation of the femoral head into the obturator foramen, where damage may be caused to the obturator nerve (**342**). Craniodorsal dislocations are more common (80% of hip dislocations), as in the cow in **338**, which shows an abnormal posture and silhouette of the left leg. In the Friesian heifer in **339** the left femoral head is dislocated upwards and forwards (craniodorsally). The bony landmarks of the hindquarters are incongruent. The left gluteal musculature is prominent owing to dorsal displacement of the greater femoral trochanter (A). Crepitus was detected on circumrotation of the femur.

338

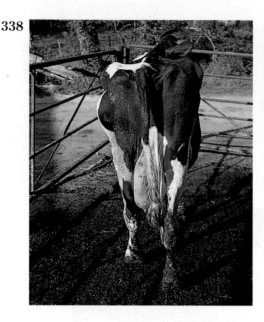

339

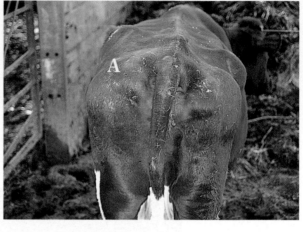

Downer cow: fractured femur

The downer cow in **340** has a right femoral midshaft fracture and related soft tissue swelling. The lower part of the right limb is deviated laterally owing to outward movement of the lower femoral shaft. The area is very painful. Such fractures do not always result in recumbency. Another femoral fracture (**341**) shows extensive soft tissue swelling and the forwards and outwards position of the leg. After one or two attempts, cattle usually abandon further efforts to stand. The underlying, nonfractured hind leg is liable to develop severe ischaemic muscle necrosis (see p.106). *Differential diagnosis*: dislocated hip (**338** & **339**).

340

341

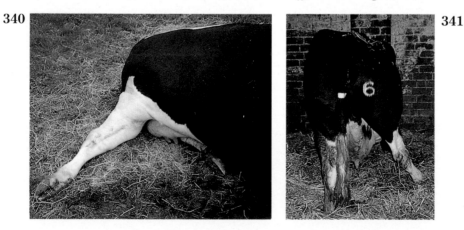

Downer cow: obturator paralysis

In **342** the abducted and symmetrical position of the hind legs is characteristic of bilateral obturator paralysis, which tends to develop after dystocia. When a newly-calved cow or heifer is walked on slippery concrete (as happened in **342**), it may slip ('do the splits'), and a dislocated hip or femoral fracture may result. Compare the degree of limb adduction in **342** with that in **343**, where there is secondary hip or femoral damage. This cow will not recover. Hobbles, applied early to the fetlock or hock region, will help to prevent excessive abduction. Another cow (**344**), partially recovered from an obturator paralysis incurred nine month previously, still abducts the right leg when walking; the left leg is normal and weight-bearing.

342 **343** **344**

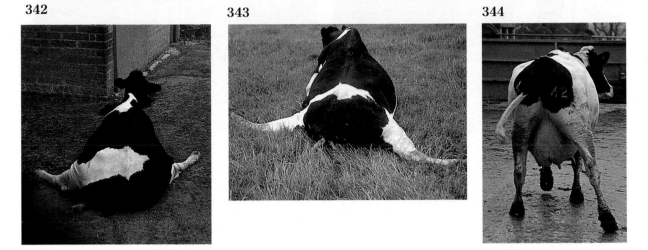

Spinal conditions

Spinal compression fracture

345

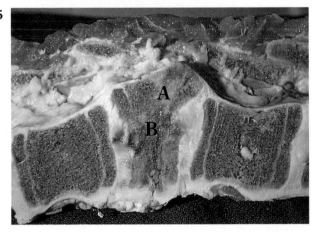

Spinal cord compression (A) (**345**) can be caused by a vertebral fracture (B). Posterior paresis had developed suddenly in this eight-month-old Holstein heifer and was probably associated with clinical rickets of several months' duration. A compression fracture had resulted in the vertebral body being slowly forced dorsally, causing kyphosis (arched back). The spinal canal became progressively stenosed and another fracture of the rachitic bone then compressed the spinal cord. Both compression fractures and septic foci in vertebral growth plates usually occur in younger cattle.

In a Friesian steer that suddenly developed kyphosis, with a discretely localised convexity of the caudal thoracic spine (**346**), rapid deterioration necessitated slaughter. Postmortem examination revealed a collapsed and infected intervertebral disc space (**347**) between the first (A) and second (B) lumbar vertebrae, resulting from a septic physitis. Deviation of the spinal canal and some spinal cord compression were evident (C).

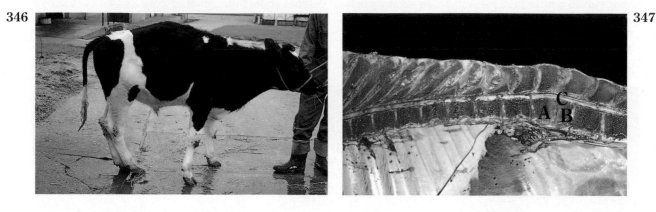

346   347

Spinal (vertebral) osteomyelitis

Osteomyelitis of the spinal vertebrae is a painful progressive disease, seen in both young and mature animals as a result of haematogenous spread. The cow in **348** had a pained expression due to vertebral abscessation, walked stiffly and was soon reluctant to stand.

Specimen **349** is a longitudinal section of the thoracolumbar spine of a six-month-old Holstein calf. Osteomyelitis affects the whole depth of a lumbar vertebral physis (growth plate). The intervertebral disc has been destroyed and the vertebral canal is stenosed. Haemorrhage is evident beneath the meninges over the stenosed cord. The infection was probably haematogenous (*Actinomyces pyogenes* was isolated).

348

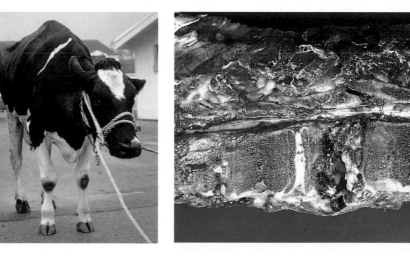

349

Spinal spondylitis

The cow in **350** has an arched thoracolumbar spine and the hind feet are placed further to the rear than normal. The right hind foot is lifted in an attempt to relieve spinal pain. Such cows often 'paddle' with the hind legs and have difficulty in rising. The condition (compare lumbar spondylosis (**336**) and spinal osteomyelitis (**348**) is a slowly progressive, aseptic process. Proliferating bone on the spinal bodies may eventually produce ankylosis (**337**).

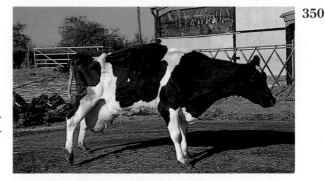

350

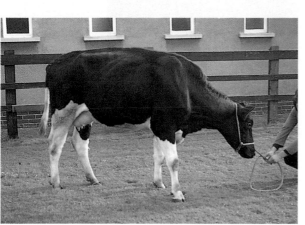

351

Cervical spinal fracture

A fracture of the fifth and sixth cervical vertebrae made the two-year-old Friesian heifer in **351** unable to lift the head and neck. A prominent dip is apparent in the dorsal cervical spine, in front of the scapula.

Sacroiliac subluxation

The wings of the ilium in the Friesian cow (**352**) are raised relative to the lumbar spine. Rectal palpation revealed the sacral promontory to be pushed backwards and depressed, resulting in a reduced dorsoventral diameter of the pelvic inlet. Subluxation occurs sporadically in cows immediately postpartum, and generally following dystocia, when it can cause temporary recumbency, the downer cow syndrome (p.106). In contrast, complete luxation (with no persisting contact of the sacrum with the ilial wings) has a poor prognosis for recovery to normal stance and locomotion. Affected cows should not be retained for breeding as the reduced pelvic inlet predisposes to dystocia.

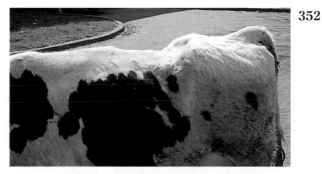

352

Tail paralysis

This Hereford bull (**353**) could not raise his tail to defecate. The prominent swelling at the tailhead (A) is an old sacrococcygeal fracture. It resulted from a fall during an attempted service of a cow, and led to compression of the coccygeal nerve supply. However, sacrococcygeal fracture does not invariably lead to nerve dysfunction, but simply to minor disfigurement, as in the two-year-old Guernsey heifer in **354**. The growing animal is especially susceptible to compression fractures of the spine and to localisation of metastatic septic foci in the growth plates of vertebral bodies.

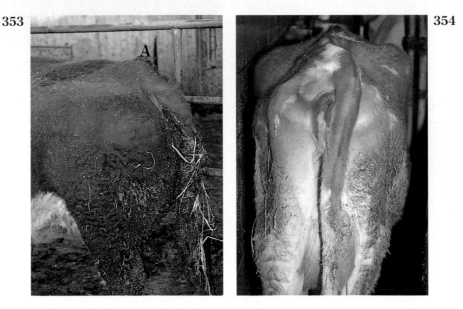

Pelvic fracture

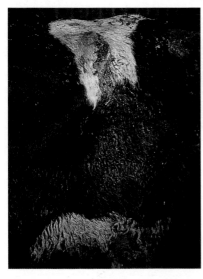

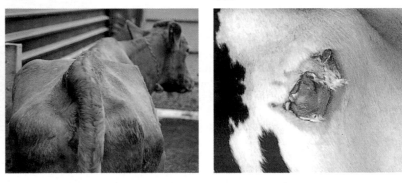

An open fracture of the left ilial wing of the cow in **355** is grossly contaminated. Such fractures arise from trauma incurred in overcrowding, when passing through doorways, or from a sudden fall on a hard surface. Most fractures of the ilial wing are closed, the fragment of bone being pulled downwards by the fascia lata, as in this Guernsey cow (**356**), where the bony prominence is absent ('dropped hip') on the right side. In other cases, the skin over the bone becomes gangrenous and sloughs (**357**). Most ilial wing fractures are nothing more than cosmetic blemishes. In contrast, ilial shaft and pubic fractures often cause severe lameness and sometimes recumbency.

Femoral fracture

The soft tissue swelling in this Simmental bull calf (**358**) overlies a femoral shaft fracture that had occurred two days previously. The stance could be confused with femoral paralysis or a hip injury such as coxofemoral luxation or femoral neck fracture. Other femoral fractures are shown in **340** & **341**.

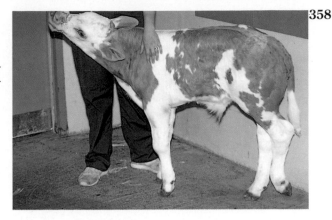

Patellar luxation

Patellar luxation may be upward or lateral, the respective clinical signs differing markedly. The right hind leg of the Holstein heifer in **359** was held in maximal extension for a few seconds and was then jerked forward. The patella was temporarily fixed above the femoral trochlea. Diagnosis (upward patellar fixation) is confirmed by the response to medial patellar desmotomy. One specific form of upward luxation and fixation occurs in growing and mature cattle, and is common among draught animals in the Indian subcontinent.

Some forms are inherited. *Differential diagnosis*: spastic paresis (**391**).

The young Holstein calf (**360**) had a flexed stifle. The patella was easily palpable, and luxated lateral to the femoral trochlea, increasing the total width of the joint. Note the accompanying gross quadriceps femoris atrophy and left hind plantigrade stance. Lateral patellar luxation is largely confined to calves less than one month old. *Differential diagnosis*: femoral paralysis (**386**).

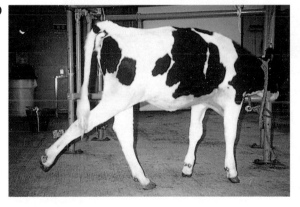

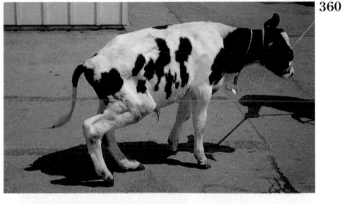

Degenerative hip arthritis

Degenerative joint disease (DJD) affects the hip and stifle more frequently than other weight-bearing joints. This hip joint of an old Hereford cow (**361**) shows the classical features of DJD: extensive erosion of articular cartilage (A), eburnation of the underlying bone (B), and a thickened joint capsule (C). The presence of blood suggests that a more recent traumatic incident had occurred after the chronic changes became established.

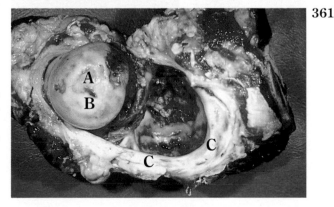

Aseptic gonitis

Aseptic or noninfectious gonitis results from trauma, and animals experience a severe and chronic lameness. The swelling in the yearling Friesian (**362**) comprises fibrosis and inflammatory fluid around the joint with secondary bone proliferation. Typically, young cattle may have a partial rupture of a collateral ligament. Some cases remain slightly lame owing to a degenerative osteoarthritis. In mature cattle (**363**) cranial cruciate ligament rupture (CrCL) is a common cause of severe stifle lameness (ruptured ligament (A)). A lateral radiograph (**364**) of the stifle joint of a similar, old, beef cow shows considerable cranial movement of the tibial articular surface on the femoral condyles (about 3 cm). A small chip is evident near the tibial eminence (A). The cranial view into the opened stifle joint in **363** shows a mere fragment of the CrCL (A), although the caudal cruciate ligament is intact (B). The medial meniscus is torn and fragmented. The medial femoral condyle shows bone loss from erosion (C), and the margin of the condyle has extensive osteophyte proliferation (D). The palpably thickened joint capsule and bony enlargement are prominent clinical signs of CrCL.

362   363   364

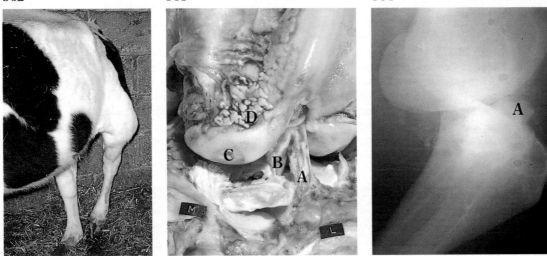

Metacarpal fractures

365   366

The Friesian calf in **365** had severe angulation following a recent distal metacarpal shaft fracture. The small amount of overlying soft tissue makes such fractures liable to perforate through the skin and become infected, hence producing osteomyelitis. Such fractures, or separation of the metacarpal physis, are very likely to occur following excessive traction in dystocia. The bilateral metacarpal shaft fractures in the Angus heifer in **366** were caused by traction on obstetrical chains placed just above the fetlocks. Note the residual scar. In this view, healing was taking place two weeks after external splintage, but note the 10–20° malalignment.

Epiphyseal separation and metacarpal fracture

The radiograph (**367**) shows a partial separation and displacement of the distal metacarpal growth plate (A), and fracture of the metaphysis (B) (Salter type II) in a neonatal calf.

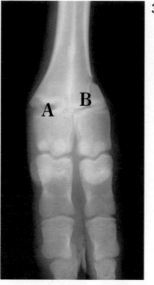

Infectious arthritis

Septic arthritis and epiphysitis

This section excludes joint ill and polyarthritis of calf-hood (see **65** in the neonatal chapter). Most forms of septic or infectious arthritis are bacterial in origin. They originate from penetrating wounds, extension from adjacent tissues (both forms being common in digital sepsis, see p.93), or by the haematogenous route.

Septic carpitis

Pressure necrosis of the skin over the carpus (knee) in a four-month-old Holstein heifer (**368**) has exposed the carpal bones. Note the peripheral epithelialisation and necrosis. A lateral radiograph of the flexed carpus (**369**) shows soft tissue swelling, bone destruction of the middle and distal rows of carpal bones, and an extensive osseous proliferative reaction (A). A sagittal section through the limb (**370**) confirms the massive tissue destruction. Infection also extends along the tendon sheaths.

368 **369** **370**

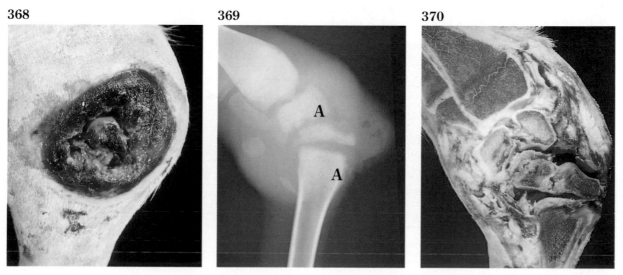

Septic arthritis of the fetlock, and tenosynovitis

The four-month-old calf in **371** has a wound (not visible) on the medial surface of the fetlock, severe septic cellulitis, tenosynovitis and arthritis leading to massive joint swelling. The fetlock joint of the Friesian cow in **372** (with flexor tendons reflected) contains inspissated pus (*Actinomyces pyogenes*), but has minimal damage to the articular cartilage. In such cases, joint infection often results from ascending digital sepsis. The longitudinal section of the metacarpus of a seven-week-old Angus heifer (**373**) shows skin necrosis, and infection has led to sepsis of the metacarpophalangeal (fetlock) joint. The skin necrosis had developed from overlong application of splints and a plaster cast (four weeks) for the immobilisation of a midshaft metacarpal fracture (A), which is seen to have healed.

371

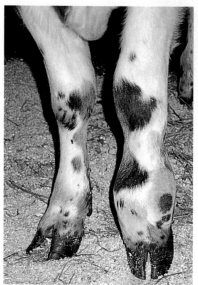

372

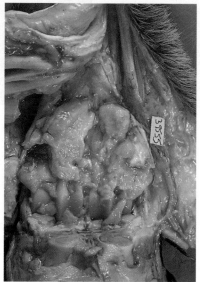

373

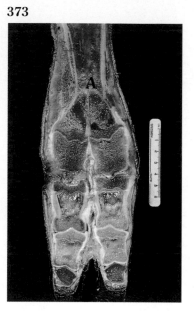

Septic arthritis of the elbow

In the 14-month-old Holstein heifer in **374**, brownish pus adheres to the joint surfaces. The articular surfaces, especially of the distal humerus, are severely eroded (A). Periarticular fibrosis is present. The usual age range for septic arthritis in calves is 1–3 months.

Chronic infectious gonitis

This old cow from Czechoslovakia (**375**) had lost a lot of weight and was in obvious pain. Long-standing degenerative and proliferative changes had caused considerable enlargement of the stifle joint. *Brucella abortus* was recovered from the synovial fluid.

374

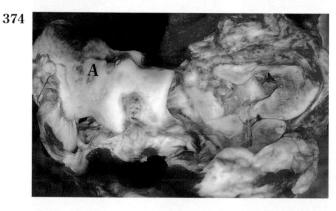

375

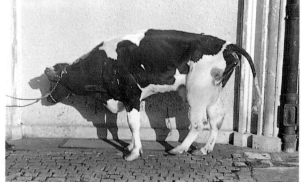

Conditions of the hock region

Hock trauma is commonly seen in confinement housing systems with inadequate bedding, and especially when the cubicle/free-stall size and design are deficient. Solid, horizontal, wooden dividing rails and vertical uprights often cause injuries. Trauma may also develop secondary to digital lameness, when cows are recumbent for long periods and have difficulty in rising. Many forms of hock swelling and injury cause little or no lameness.

Tarsal bursitis and cellulitis

376

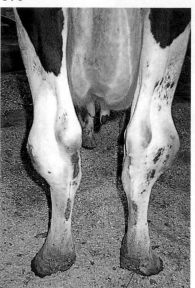

377

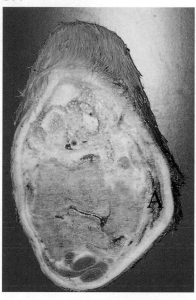

378

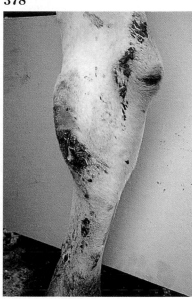

Lateral swellings over the subcutaneous bursae of both hocks (also called cellulitis) are common in cattle housed on concrete (**376**). Carpal hygroma (**390**) causes a similar foreleg problem. The hair loss results from chronic abrasion. A horizontal section through an affected hock (**377**) shows a discrete discoloured cavity (A) lined with granulation tissue. The synovia-like fluid is sterile. The majority of cases are not infected. An outward deviation of the digits (cow-hocked) often contributes to the development of tarsal bursitis.

Occasionally, the skin barrier is broken and the wound becomes infected and discharges pus (**378**). The swelling then tends to be more diffuse than in aseptic bursitis, and marked pain and lameness result. In another cow the left hock is very swollen and an area on the plantar surface is necrotic and septic (**379**). The injury resulted from a puncture wound which introduced infection into the subcutaneous tissues. Although such affected animals do become very lame, this animal recovered after antibiotic therapy.

379

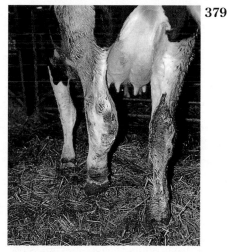

Medial tarsal hygroma

The bilateral swelling in **380** is fluctuating, painless, and causes only slight mechanical lameness from its size. The condition is uncommon and the aetiology is unknown.

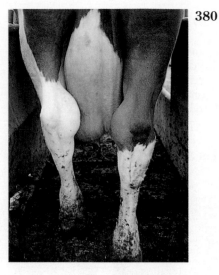

380

Tenosynovitis of the tarsal sheath ('capped hock')

A firm swelling surrounds the point of the hock of this three-year-old Holstein cow (**381**) and extends distally towards the tibiotarsal joint. Six months previously, the cow had fallen through a metal grid, sustaining an open wound involving the medial aspect of the tarsal sheath. Sepsis resulted, but the wound eventually healed with fibrosis.

381

Gastrocnemius trauma

Trauma to the gastrocnemius muscle—tendon group arises sporadically from struggling, as when a cow with hypocalcaemia (milk fever) attempts to stand following a period of recumbency. Rare cases are associated with vitamin D deficiency and aphosphorosis. The prognosis is generally hopeless, except in young animals, where external support may permit slow healing by fibrosis. Two manifestations of gastrocnemius rupture are shown. The first (**382**) shows a dropped hock and swelling of the gastrocnemius muscle belly in a Shorthorn heifer.

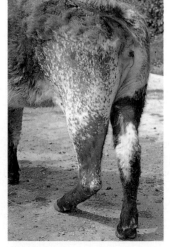

382

The Ayrshire cow in **383** has a complete bilateral rupture, cannot stand, and bears weight on the plantar surfaces of the hock and metatarsus. Another form of gastrocnemius injury is traumatic transection, as shown in the two-year-old Friesian heifer in **384**. This injury arises from a slicing action and can be very severe. The wound is invariably infected. Since both gastrocnemius and superficial flexor tendons are involved, weightbearing is made impossible.

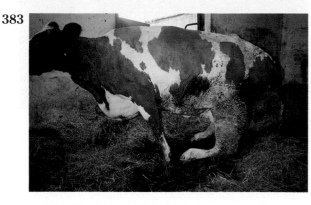

383

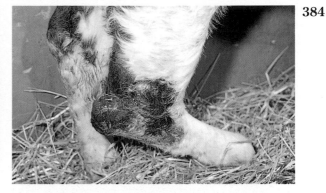

384

Peripheral paralyses

One form of peripheral paralysis (obturator) has already been illustrated in the context of the downer cow syndrome (**342**). The four other types of nerve damage, that are illustrated below, do not often result in this syndrome.

Sciatic paralysis

Left sciatic paralysis resulted from the accidental (iatrogenic) perineural injection of an antibiotic solution into the deep gluteal region of this Angus heifer (**385**). Long-acting antibiotic preparations are commonly implicated. Sciatic paralysis occasionally develops following prolonged recumbency resulting from parturient paresis. Severe ischaemic muscle necrosis is evident around the damaged nerve (see downer cow, p.106).

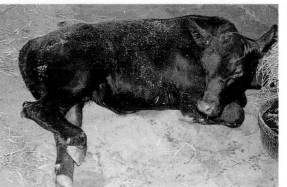

385

Femoral paralysis

The flexed stifle cannot be extended to allow weightbearing, owing to dysfunction of the quadriceps group in this four-day-old Simmental calf (**386**). Skin sensation was absent over part of the medial aspect of the thigh. A secondary lateral patellar luxation is sometimes present (**360**). A hollowed-out appearance of the quadriceps muscle (atrophy) is seen after about 7–10 days. Neonatal cases are the most common and their pathogenesis is often unclear. Foetal hyperextension caused by excessive traction during delivery, muscular compression and ischaemic anoxia may account for the clinical signs.

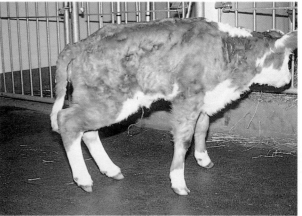

386

Peroneal paralysis

Peroneal paralysis is a common postpartum injury. The stance of the six-year-old Holstein in **387** resulted from paralysis of the hock flexors and digital extensors. Paresis or paralysis may persist for days or weeks, or, occasionally, indefinitely. The peroneal nerve is most susceptible to damage over the lateral surface of the stifle joint, and injury with subsequent paralysis is therefore seen following recumbency on a hard surface.

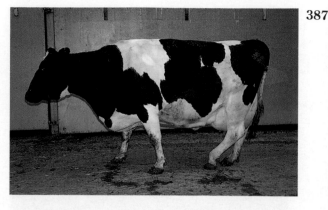

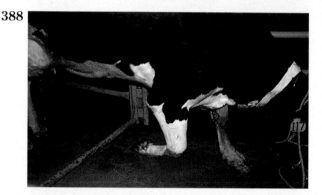

Radial paralysis

This mature Holstein cow (**388**) shows a dropped elbow, a flexed carpus and fetlock, and an inability to bear weight. The cow had been maintained under general anaesthesia, in right lateral recumbency on a padded table for two and a half hours. Paralysis was immediately evident on standing and the gait was normal two days later. *Differential diagnosis*: humeral fracture.

Brachial plexus injury

The elbow of the Friesian heifer in **389** was dropped, but the forelimb could be advanced for some limited weightbearing. This injury can result from severe abduction of the forelimb. Some radial paralysis (the radial nerve being one component of the plexus) was present.

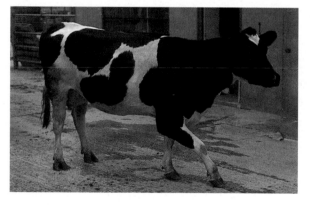

Miscellaneous locomotor conditions

Carpal hygroma

Carpal hygromata rarely reach the size seen in the right leg of this old Friesian cow (**390**). They are usually bilateral, contain thin serum-like material, and cause little or no lameness. Like tarsal bursitis (see **376**), carpal hygromata result from repeated contusions on hard surfaces (concrete) in poorly designed housing, or from brucellosis.

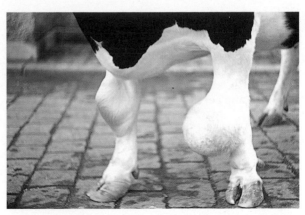

Spastic paresis ('Elso heel')

In this six-month-old Friesian heifer (**391**) the left hock is overextended, and the gastrocnemius tendon and muscle were tense on palpation. This inherited condition, sporadically seen in both dairy and beef breeds, affects one or both hind limbs, producing a progressive disability that starts at 2–9 months old. Surgical correction can be performed, but is not recommended in breeding animals. *Differential diagnosis*: dorsal patellar luxation, joint ill, gonitis, localised spinal trauma or space-occupying lesion.

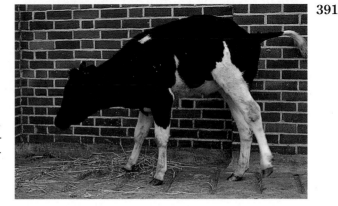

Hip dysplasia

The yearling Hereford bull in **392** has severe atrophy of the hindquarters. The forefeet are placed caudally and the hindfeet cranially to increase the proportion of weight borne by the forequarters. The acetabulum of another Hereford bull (**393**) shows the extensive cartilaginous erosion and areas of bone loss that result from this degenerative process. Hip dysplasia is a progressive and probably inherited, bilateral, degenerative joint disease, seen in several beef breeds including the Aberdeen Angus and the Hereford. The clinical signs start at 2–18 months old.

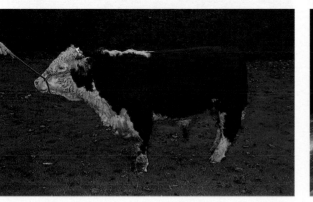

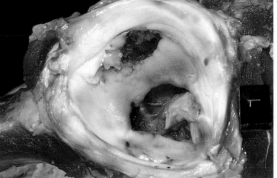

Osteochondrosis dissecans (OCD)

OCD occasionally causes a degenerative and aseptic joint problem of unknown aetiology in young, fast-growing beef cattle. The opened joints of a yearling Angus crossbred steer (**394**) that had chronic, bilaterally enlarged shoulder joints, leading to lameness and poor growth, show loss of cartilage and subchondral bone (A), and periarticular fibrosis (B).

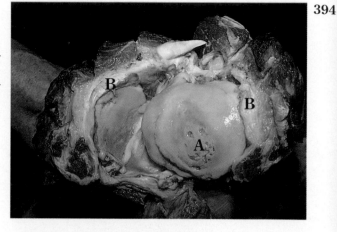

Septic myositis (popliteal abscess)

The massive swelling seen in the right thigh of this two-year-old Simmental bull (**395**) caused a moderate lameness. The lighter area had been clipped for exploratory puncture. The swelling contained 12 litres of pus (isolate: *Actinomyces pyogenes*). For a further discussion, see popliteal abscess (**118**).

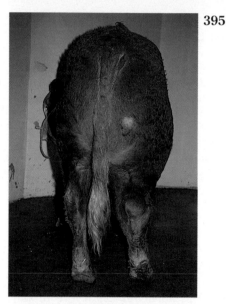

Rupture of the ventral serrate muscle

The right scapula of the mature Flemish Maas–Rijn–Ijssel cow in **396** projects above the thoracic spine owing to the rupture of the ventral serrate and subscapular muscles. The scapula returns to its normal anatomical position when the leg is not bearing weight. In mature cattle the aetiology is probably chronic muscle degeneration and atrophy.

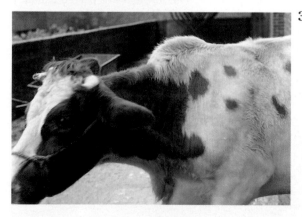

White muscle disease

In fattening beef cattle (**397**), in which the condition is also termed 'flying scapula', muscular dystrophy and white muscle disease resulting from a combined vitamin E and selenium deficiency, may be involved in the rupture of the same muscles as in **396**. The heart of a calf with white muscle disease (**398**) has extensive pale greyish areas on the epicardium. This pallor typically extends into the myocardium, and there may also be endothelial plaques. The cardiac shape is globular following chronic hypertrophy. White muscle lesions are usually bilateral. They are seen in skeletal muscle and in the diaphragm, and result from peroxide-induced muscle-fibre necrosis following calcium deposition.

397

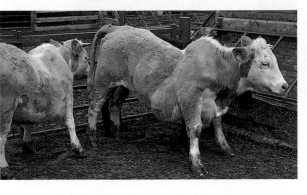

398

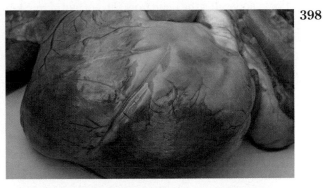

Foreign body around the metatarsus

In **399** a piece of wire is being removed from a characteristic, deep, circumferential, granulating wound of the metatarsal soft tissues. The two-year-old Limousin bull was moderately lame and recovered rapidly.

399

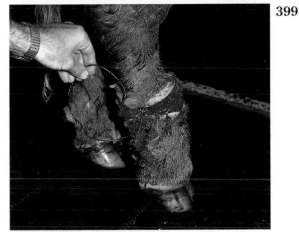

Distal limb gangrene: traumatic origin

In **400** a clear line demarcates the dead from the healthy skin. The Holstein cow had caught her leg at the metacarpal level in a stanchion chain, and was found recumbent the following morning, with the chain still in place. A few days later the skin was dry and painless. It sloughed three weeks later, together with the distal soft tissues and hoof horn capsule, necessitating euthanasia.

400

Fescue foot gangrene

Fescue foot is caused by an ergot-like toxin, consumed by cattle grazing certain endophyte-infested strains of tall fescue grasses in many states of the USA, as well as in New Zealand, Italy and Australia.

In the 11-month-old Hereford steer in **401**, the dark areas of skin on the hind pasterns are dry gangrene. A sharply-defined oblique line (A) extending over the fetlock, separates the dead from the normal skin. Skin has also separated from the coronary band to expose infected subcutis (B). The upper (right) limb shows a pink area where the gangrenous skin has sloughed. The ear tips and tail may also become gangrenous. *Differential diagnosis*: ergotism (**402**), frostbite (**123**), trauma (**400**) and salmonellosis (**50**).

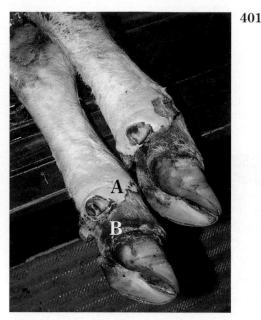

401

Ergot gangrene

Gangrene of the extremities resulting from the ingestion of ergot-infested cereals and other feeds is a worldwide problem. The clinical features resemble fescue foot (**401**). The feet and tail tip are affected in the yearling heifer in **402**. Gangrenous skin is sloughing from the left metatarsal region, and a similar line of demarcation is seen in the right leg. The distal 25 cm of the tail is twisted, moist and gangrenous.

More advanced changes in the feet are shown in **403**. The left foot has almost sloughed at the pastern, and the distal third of the tail is detached. Ergotism results from ingestion of the parasitic fungus *Claviceps purpurea* on hay, grain or seeded pastures. *Differential diagnosis*: fescue foot (**401**), frostbite (**123**), trauma (**400**), and salmonellosis (**50**).

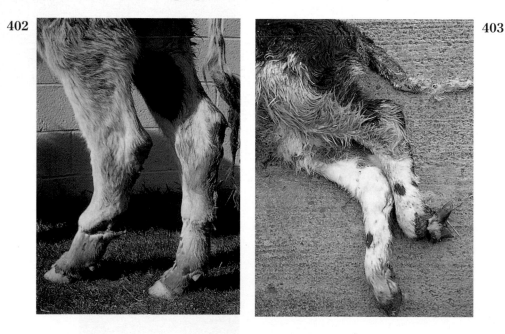

402

403

Hyaena disease

This severely affected, three-and-a-half-year-old French Friesian cow (**404**) has a hyaena-like silhouette, with underdevelopment of the hindquarters. Calves are normal at birth, and manifest the initial signs of the disease at 6–10 months. Compared with a normal tibia of a two-year-old animal (**405**, left), the tibia of an affected individual (22 months) is considerably shortened, although the width and articular surface area are comparable. The condition is thought to result from a bone dysplasia.

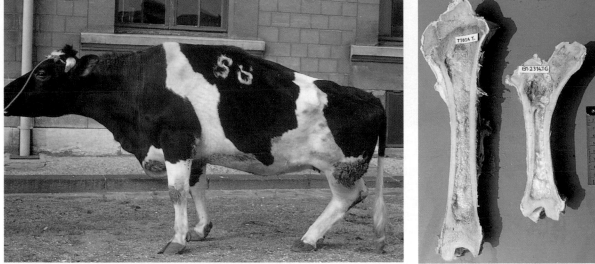

404

405

Deficiency diseases

Rickets

Rickets, caused by a calcium, phosphorus or vitamin D deficiency, involves a failure of calcification of osteoid and cartilage. Swelling and pain generally involve all the major limb joints.

In the six-month old Holstcin hcifer in **406** the fetlock is enlarged due to widening of the distal metacarpal physis. The articular surfaces are normal. The calf is lame. *Differential diagnosis*: copper deficiency (**413**) and epiphysitis. See also spinal compression fracture (**345**).

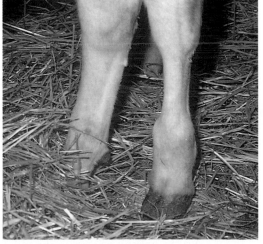

406

Phosphorus deficiency (osteomalacia)

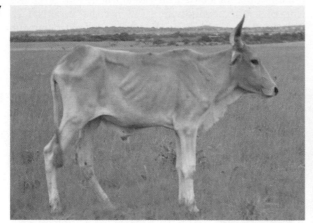

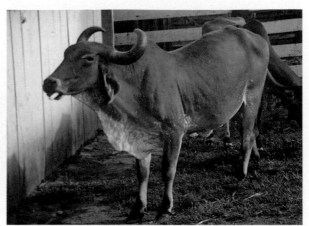

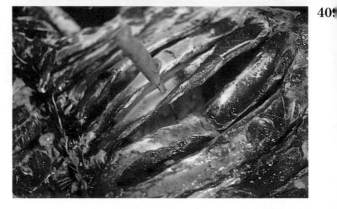

Phosphorus deficiency is the most common mineral deficiency worldwide. Affected cattle are unthrifty, have a poor appetite and walk stiffly. The Brazilian steer in **407** is stunted, extremely emaciated, and walked with great difficulty. The local term for this severe aphosphorosis is 'entreva'. The Brazilian Zebu (Gir) cow (**408**) is eating a bone, demonstrating pica; other bones litter the ground. This habit may result in botulism (**687**). A carcase of a phosphorus-deficient animal from the Australian outback has multiple fractured ribs that are so soft they can easily be cut with a knife (**409**). A phosphorus deficiency in young cattle causes rickets (**406**) with slow growth and joint deformities. The easiest and cheapest prophylaxis is the supply of a phosphatic mineral supplement in troughs or boxes protected from the rain. *Differential diag-*

nosis: other mineral deficiencies, e.g., calcium, copper and cobalt, and starvation.

Copper deficiency (hypocuprosis)

The crossbred Hereford heifer in **410** is unthrifty and has enlarged fetlocks and a characteristic brownish tinge to the hair coat. The loss of hair pigment may produce a 'spectacled' appearance, as seen in the crossbred Charolais calf in **411**. (The Hereford also has lice.) Bone fragility and anaemia are other clinical features. The Brazilian cows in **412** show poor growth, poor hair coat and loss of pigment. The fetlock joint enlargement (**413**) is due to widening and irregularity of the metacarpal physes, as seen in the radiographs (**414**) of an affected animal (left) compared with a normal animal (right). Similar radiographic changes are seen in the digits. Other cattle may become stunted, developing bowed legs, contracted tendons and kyphosis. Excluding phosphorus deficiency, a deficiency of copper may be the most severe

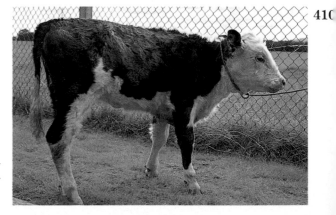

mineral limitation to grazing livestock in extensive tropical regions. *Differential diagnosis:* aphosphorosis(**407**), rickets(**406**), and cobalt deficiency(**416**).

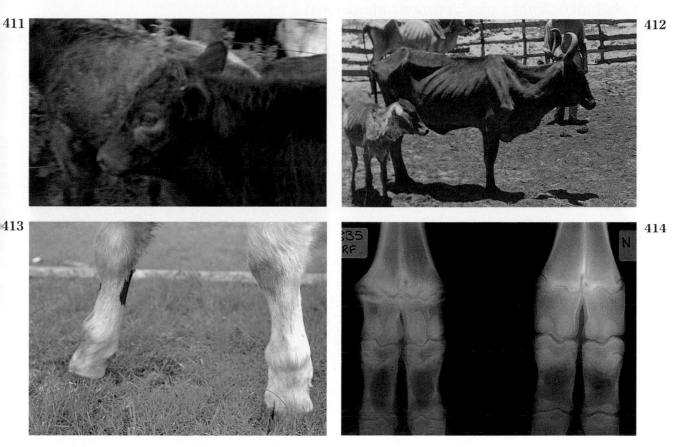

Manganese deficiency

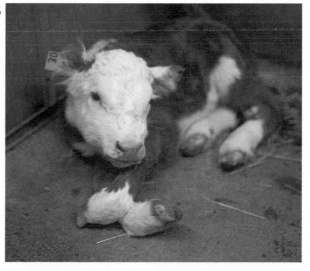

This Hereford neonate (**415**) cannot stand owing to a congenital twisting and flexion of the enlarged fetlock joints. Various other skeletal abnormalities are also present. These changes resulted from a severe manganese deficiency in the dam during gestation. In a 100-head Hereford herd in Canada, of the 5–10% of calves that were born with abnormalities, this calf was among the most severely affected. Following external splintage, many calves recovered from tendon contracture.

Cobalt deficiency ('pine', enzootic marasmus)

The Brazilian Zebu cattle are depressed, emaciated, eat little and have a poor hair coat (**416**). They are also anaemic. Visual evidence of cobalt deficiency is non-specific, resembling the signs of semistarvation. Young animals are more susceptible. Diagnosis may ultimately rest on the response to cobalt supplementation. *Differential diagnosis*: aphosphorosis (osteomalacia)(**407**), hypocuprosis (**410**), parasitism and low feed intake.

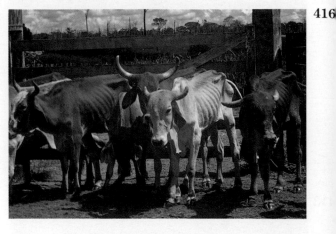
416

8 Ocular disorders

Introduction

Disorders of the eye are relatively easily seen and photographed. The disorders may be congenital, nutritional, infectious, traumatic or neoplastic in origin. Examples of each are illustrated. Some conditions, for example, infectious bovine keratoconjunctivitis (IBK), occur worldwide, and may be a significant cause of economic loss. Pain associated with the active phase of disease restricts feeding and leads to weight loss. If sight is lost, affected animals are less able to forage, particularly under extensive ranch conditions, and they are more susceptible to predators.

Congenital disorders

Although congenital abnormalities are, by definition, present at birth, some may not be recognised until the calf is much older. Strabismus (squint) is a typical example. Congenital disorders may be genetic, and therefore inherited, or they may be caused by environmental factors. Some abnormalities have more than one cause. For example, congenital cataract may be inherited, or it may have been caused by maternal BVD infection during pregnancy. The cause of many abnormalities is unknown. Congenital disorders in organs other than the eye are described in Chapter 1.

Anophthalmia (anophthalmos); microphthalmia (microphthalmos)

The two examples illustrate true anophthalmia, in that there is total absence of the globe. Microphthalmia is defined as reduced dimensions of the eye. The left eye of the Guernsey heifer in **417** has a small orbit and there is no evidence of the globe. Note that the entire orbit appears collapsed and smaller, compared with the normal right eye. The close-up of the Gloucester calf (**418**), in which both eyes were totally absent, shows an intact third eyelid and the orbit lined with conjunctiva.

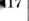**17**

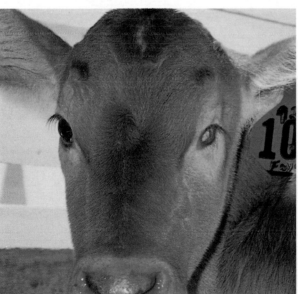

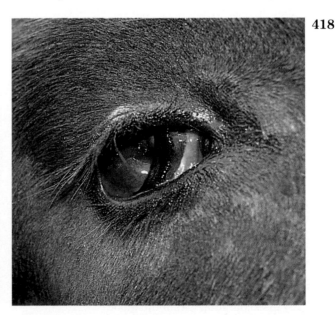418

Congenital cataract

Both eyes of the four-day-old Hereford crossbred calf in **419** were affected and the animal was totally blind. In other animals, only one eye may be affected, or the cataract may not cause total loss of vision. Congenital cataract is not normally progressive. Even blind cattle can be reared in confinement systems. They quickly learn to remain within the group, although handling can be difficult. Congenital cataract may be inherited, or may result from the teratogenic effects of maternal BVD infection during early/mid pregnancy. **420** shows a congenital nuclear cataract in a young Friesian calf.

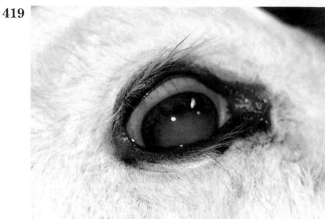

419

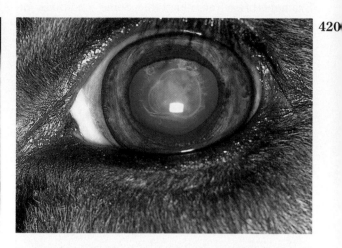

420

Coloboma

A coloboma is a congenital cleft caused by failure of the embryonic optic fissure to close. It can occur in the eyelids, iris, lens, or, as shown in **421**, the retina. Note the pale area devoid of functional retinal cells. The condition is inherited in certain breeds of cattle (e.g., Charolais), but vision is not normally impaired.

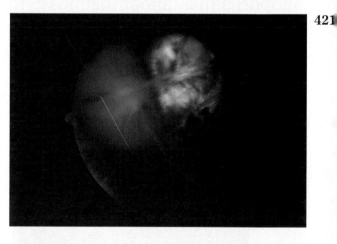

421

Strabismus ('squint')

Strabismus may be convergent, when the visual axes of the eyes converge more than is required for normal vision, or divergent. **422** shows divergent strabismus in the left eye of a Guernsey heifer. Exophthalmos with strabismus may be inherited, although it is often unnoticed until 6–9 months old. Sometimes known as 'wall eye', this term more commonly refers to a blue-grey discolouration within the globe.

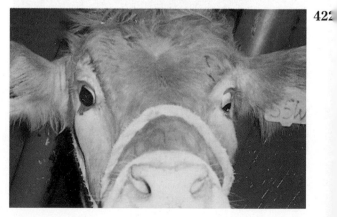

422

Neonatal corneal opacity

In the stillborn Charolais calf in **423**, a reduction in intraocular pressure led to cloudiness in the cornea and indicated that the calf had died at least 12 hours before birth. The eyeball is slightly sunken in the socket.

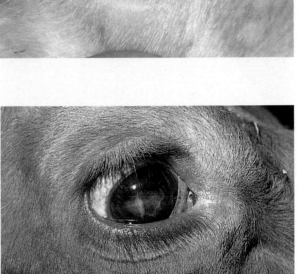

Acquired cataract

Note the two large synechiae (adhesions of the iris to the cornea), and the opacity and wrinkling of the lens in the Guernsey cow in **424**. Cataracts may be secondary to inflammatory processes within the eye, when they can be progressive. In contrast, congenital cataracts (**419**) are not normally progressive.

Vitamin A deficiency

In young growing animals, vitamin A deficiency blindness is associated with stenosis of the optic foramen and consequent pressure on the optic nerve. The pupil becomes dilated and degenerative changes may be seen on the retina (**425**). The optic disc is pale and enlarged, with indistinct margins (papilloedema). White mottling of the nontapetal area suggests chorioretinal mottling. The steer was blind. (The diet had been barley straw, rolled barley and, occasionally, poor-quality hay.)

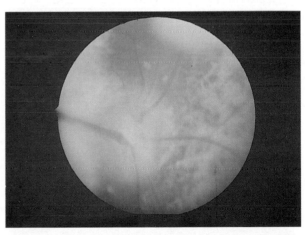

Conjunctivitis

Mild conjunctivitis is seen clinically as epiphora. Typically, a wet, black-stained facial area radiates from the medial canthus. More advanced cases (**426**) show a degree of photophobia. Purulent conjunctivitis (**427**) may also be seen. Caused by a variety of infections and irritants, conjunctivitis and epiphora commonly occur in association with other diseases, for example, calf pneumonia (**233**), IBR (**222**), IBK (**428**) and ocular foreign body (**438**).

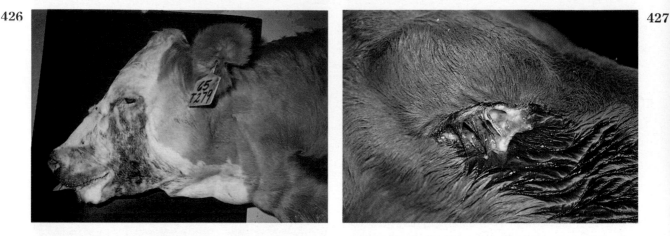

426
427

Infectious bovine keratoconjunctivitis (IBK, infectious ophthalmia, 'New Forest disease' or 'pinkeye')

A bacterial infection caused by *Moraxella bovis*, IBK produces conjunctivitis, keratitis and corneal ulceration. In mild cases, corneal ulceration may not be apparent. Bright sunlight, dry, dusty and irritant conditions, flies, and a tight stocking density are all predisposing factors. Typically the ulcer is in the centre of the cornea (compare ocular foreign body (**438**), where it is peripheral) and may be superficial or erode deeply into the stroma (**428**). The condition is very painful, leading to photophobia, blepharospasm and epiphora. Note the encrustation of the lower lids due to lacrimation. Very early corneal vascularisation (A) can be seen in **428**, as well as early pannus formation. The pupil (B) is miotic. Later stages (**429**) develop corneal opacity due to increased intraocular pressure. The bright red rim of pannus (A), progressing from the corneoscleral junction to fill the ulcer, is clearly evident.

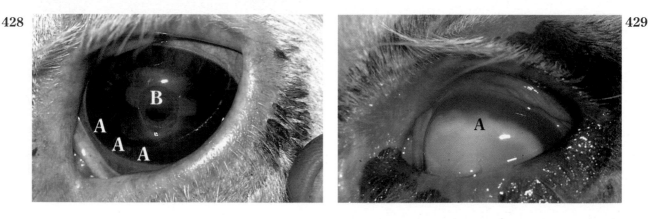

428
429

This will regress when healing is complete. Pannus formation does not occur with shallow, superficial lesions, where the ulcer is seen in a localised area of corneal opacity (**430**). If corneal rupture does not occur, healing may be complete, or may leave a small corneal scar (A), as seen towards the medial canthus in **431**. Partial sight has been regained. The circular plaque (B) on the cornea is an artefact caused by flash photography.

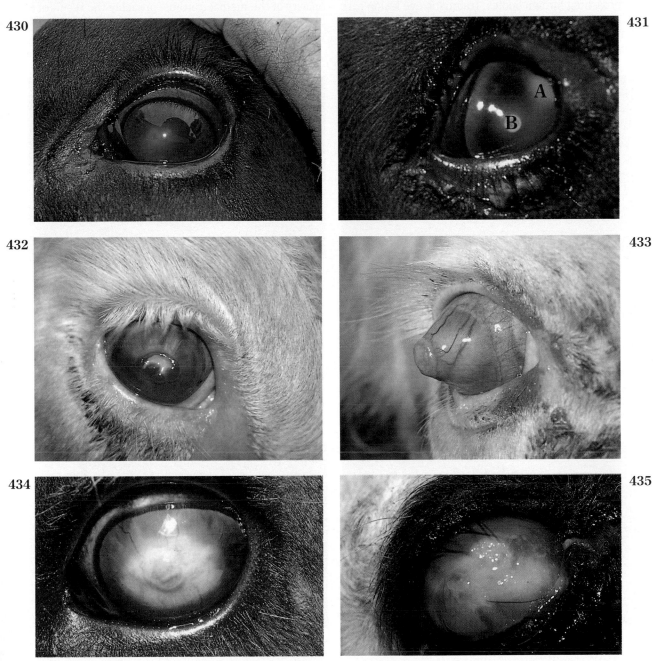

Deep ulcers may perforate through to the aqueous. In **432**, tissue from the iris plugs the ruptured ulcer and can be seen as a red ring protruding from the surface of the cornea. This is a staphyloma. More advanced cases (**433**) lose their red appearance and some may eventually heal, but they leave an opaque, scarred cornea (**434**) and glaucoma from impaired drainage of the aqueous humour.

Secondary infection of the eye (**435**) (endophthalmitis) leads to pus in the anterior chamber (hypopyon). The eyeball is protruding, there is pannus formation, and the cornea is white and irregular. Sight has now been permanently lost.

Ocular trauma

Although the eye is well protected within the bony orbit and by the rapid reflex closure of the lids to approaching foreign bodies, traumatic eye lesions are common, particularly those due to incoming objects. Irritation due to dust or ultraviolet light may produce keratitis and conjunctivitis. The Guernsey cow in **436** has a congested scleral conjunctiva (seen below the upper eyelid), an indistinct pupil, and mild corneal opacity at the medial canthus, probably the result of a blow. The four-day-old Jersey calf in **437** shows marked scleral haemorrhage resulting from dystocia.

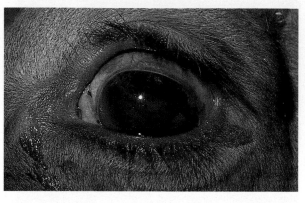

436

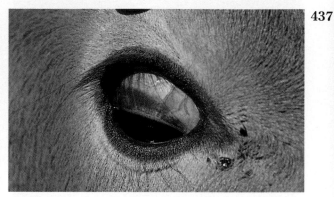

437

Ocular foreign body

Grass seeds or other plant material may become lodged in the conjunctiva and, as the eyeball moves, repeatedly traumatise the area to produce erosion and ulceration. Cattle reaching up to feed from overhead hay racks are particularly at risk. In **438** a small fragment of plant material (A) is embedded in the corneal surface near the lateral canthus. Note the surrounding early peripheral keratitis and corneal opacity. Keratitis with early corneal ulceration is seen in the more advanced case in **439**. Most of the foreign body is lodged in the lateral canthus, with one small fragment protruding across the cornea.

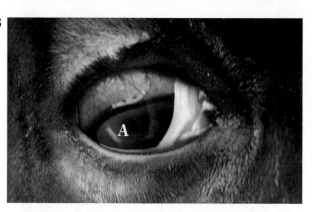

438

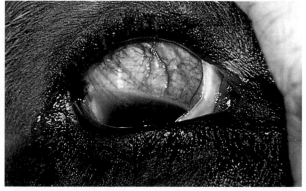

439

Prolapse of the eyeball (proptosis)

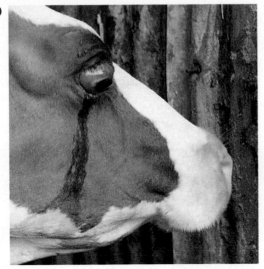

440

Prolapse of the eyeball is an infrequent condition caused by trauma to the head. In the Ayrshire cow in **440**, note the congested and oedematous sclera and the eyeball protruding beyond the lids. Repulsion and surgical fixation resulted in a successful recovery.

Eyelid laceration

Lacerations of the lower eyelids are fairly common. They are often caused by an animal rubbing and catching its eyelid on projections from troughs, buildings or fragments of wire. In the Angus heifer in **441**, the lower lid injury near the lateral canthus was sustained several days previously and was healing well.

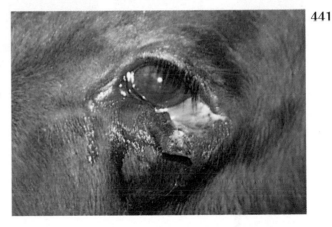

441

Hyphaema

442

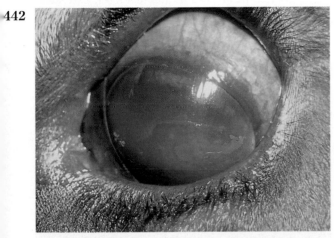

Hyphaema is haemorrhage of blood into the anterior chamber. In **442** note the superficial dry keratitis and the fresh blood beneath the cornea. Although hyphaema is usually traumatic, this case was due to sepsis. (See also bracken poisoning, **699**).

Bovine iritis (uveitis, iridocyclitis)

Bovine iritis has been associated with *Listeria* infection from the feeding of big-bale silage. Early cases (**443**) show an enlarged and wrinkled iris, leading to a central miotic pupil. Near the lateral canthus is a white endothelial plaque on the inner surface of the cornea (Descemet's membrane), with corneal opacity and early pannus formation. As the condition progresses (**444**), pannus develops circumferentially (A), with increasing corneal discolouration and opacity (B). In severe cases (**445**) the endothelial plaques produce a very irregular surface on the cornea and cause complete blindness. However, even such advanced cases may recover following subconjunctival anti-inflammatory and antibiotic treatment.

443   **444**   **445**

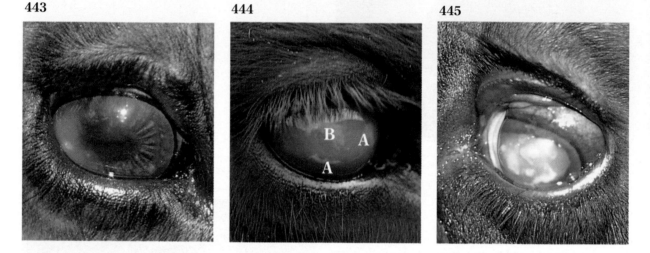

Neoplastic conditions

Malignancy of the third eyelid (membrana nictitans) and the globe is common in cattle worldwide. Lymphosarcomas may occur within the globe itself, or in the orbit, leading to prolapse of the globe. Papillomas have been reported occasionally.

Squamous cell carcinoma

Squamous cell carcinoma (SCC) is the most common ocular neoplasm of cattle, and is seen particularly in white-headed cattle, such as the Hereford, and other breeds with little pigmentation around the eye. The disease is associated with ultraviolet light. Common sites for SCC include the lower lid, the third eyelid and the corneoscleral junction of the globe. The Hereford bull in **446** has SCC at several points along the eyelids (A), a greyish plaque, 10 mm in diameter, extending over the cornea from the corneoscleral junction (B), and early SCC in the third eyelid (C). In the Guernsey cow in **447**, pink, neoplastic tissue protrudes from the

446   **447**

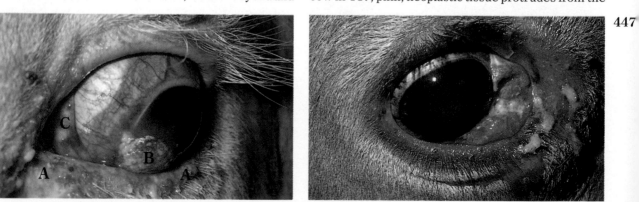

third eyelid (membrana nictitans) at the medial canthus. There is a secondary, superficial, purulent infection. Early lesions are easily removed, but in neglected cases, ten per cent will eventually metastasise to the regional lymph nodes, and a small proportion to the lungs, as in **448**. The multiple irregular pale areas are tumour tissue.

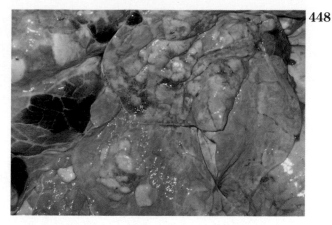

448

Lymphosarcoma

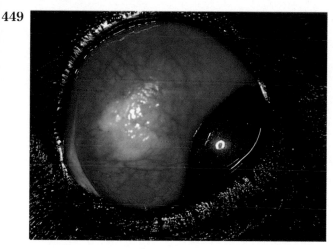

449

In **449** a large neoplastic mass has produced a smooth, red, bulbous enlargement of the conjunctiva, compressing the eyeball towards the medial canthus (right). Lymphosarcoma is the most common orbital tumour and causes progressive exophthalmos. The tumour is almost invariably present at other sites.

Papilloma of the third eyelid

In **450** the lesion is attached to the third eyelid by a 'stalk' and has a very irregular keratinised surface. It is much less common than a squamous cell carcinoma, and is easy to remove surgically.

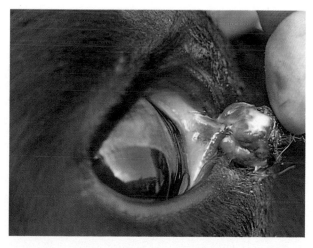

450

9 Nervous Disorders

Introduction

The nervous diseases discussed in this chapter are those in which nervous signs comprise the major part of the clinical syndrome. Consequently, a wide range of aetiology is covered including nutritional conditions (e.g., cerebrocortical necrosis), metabolic disorders (e.g., hypomagnesaemia), bacterial and viral infections (e.g., listeriosis and rabies), parasites (e.g., *Coenurus cerebralis*), physical and traumatic incidents (lightning stroke and electrocution) and miscellaneous conditions of uncertain aetiology (e.g., bovine spongiform encephalopathy). However, other diseases with significant clinical nervous signs may be featured elsewhere. Examples include tetanus (**685**), botulism (**687**) and lead poisoning (**726**).

Nervous conditions may be difficult to appreciate in 'still' photographs, since their clinical assessment is based on changes in behaviour, movement, gait and stance. As such, an understanding of the normal animal is extremely important. Where problems of recognition occur, the text has been expanded in an attempt to describe those changes that cannot be photographed.

Cerebrocortical necrosis (polioencephalomalacia)

Cerebrocortical necrosis (CCN) is a thiamine-related condition, induced by products of abnormal ruminal fermentation (thiaminases). It is seen most commonly in calves that are 2–6 months old, often following a dietary change. In the Friesian calf in **451**, note the pronounced opisthotonos, the rotation of the eye to expose the sclera, and the extensor spasm of the front legs. Postmortem lesions (**452**) are normally symmetrical and occur in the frontal, occipital and parietal lobes. Congestion and yellow degeneration of the cortical grey matter (A) is seen, typically at the junction of the white and grey matter, particularly on the left and right extremities. Affected brains will fluoresce blue-green under ultraviolet light.

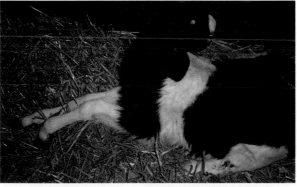

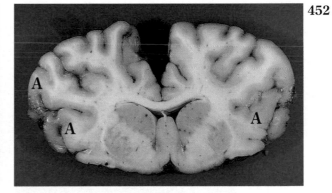

Metabolic diseases

Metabolic diseases are included in this chapter, since many of their presenting clinical signs are behavioural or nervous. Typically, they occur when homeostasis has been extended beyond physiological limits. Four conditions are illustrated: hypomagnesaemia, hypocalcaemia, acetonaemia and fatty liver syndrome.

Hypomagnesaemia ('grass staggers', 'grass tetany').

The Friesian cow in **453** fell and developed extensor spasm when being brought in for milking. Note the 'staring' eye, dilated pupil, frothing at the mouth and sweaty coat. In **454** the crossbred cow from Queensland, Australia, shows similar eye changes. The head and the hind legs are in extensor spasm. Violent paddling movements of the forelegs and head have result-ed in loss of foliage, exposing the bare earth. Precipitated by stress and seen especially in temperate climates, the condition is induced by grazing magnesium-deficient or high potassium pastures, and other pastures where magnesium uptake is poor. Concurrent hypocalcaemia may be an exacerbating factor.

453

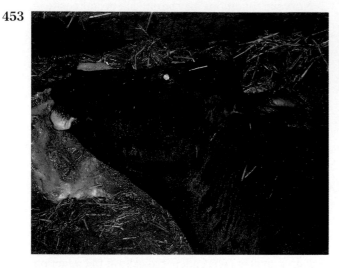

454

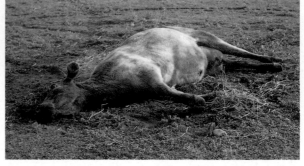

Hypocalcaemia ('milk fever', post-parturient paresis)

Hypocalcaemia (**455**) occurs typically in older cows immediately pre- or post-calving. Affected animals are unable to rise owing to lack of muscle power and poor nerve function. Note also the protruding anal sphincter (due to accumulation of faeces in the rectum, and increased intra-abdominal pressure), slight ruminal bloat (ruminal atony) and the typical 'S-bend' in the neck. This is thought to be a self-righting response, as the animal attempts to avoid full lateral recumbency. Some affected cows lie with their head resting on their flank (**456**).

455

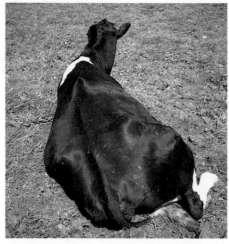

456

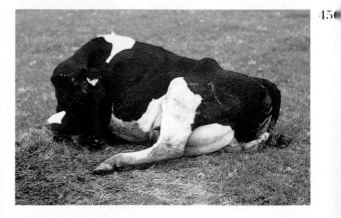

140

Nervous acetonaemia (ketosis, 'slow fever')

457

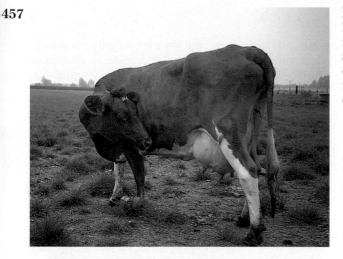

Nervous acetonaemia is an intoxication by circulating ketone bodies and is associated with an energy deficit in early lactation. Typical clinical signs are anorexia and lethargy (hence 'slow fever'), although some cases develop nervous signs such as compulsive licking, salivation, biting flanks (as seen in the Guernsey cow in (**457**) or even maniacal behaviour.

Fatty liver syndrome (fat cow syndrome)

Fatty liver syndrome is related to ketosis and is seen especially in overfat cows that are fed an energy–deficient diet after calving. Many cows show no precise clinical signs. More advanced cases develop anorexia and 'star–gazing', as in the Jersey cow in **458**, progressing to terminal recumbency.

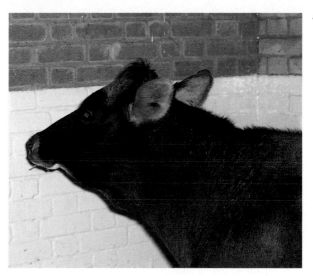

458

Bacterial infections

Listeriosis ('circling disease')

A bacterial infection caused by *Listeria monocytogenes*, listeriosis is a meningoencephalitis that produces pyrexia, dullness, blindness and a unilateral facial nerve paralysis, leading to prolapse of the tongue (**459**) and drooping of the ears. The organism is ubiquitous, being found in most wildlife. Compulsive circling towards the affected side (**460**) is also often seen, and abortions may occur, but they are usually not concurrent with nervous signs. The disease is associated with cold weather and silage feeding. *Differential diagnosis*: rabies (**478**), acute lead poisoning (**726**), CCN (**451**), botulism (**687**), bacterial meningitis (**465**), viral encephalitis and pituitary abscess (**464**).

459
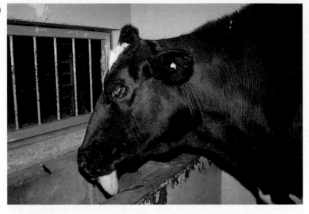

46(
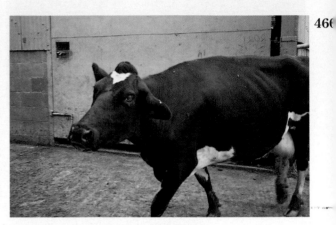

Middle ear infection (otitis media)

In middle ear infections, the head is typically held to one side, as in the young Friesian bull in **461**. However, the animal remained alert, continued feeding and was not pyrexic. The eyelid is swollen owing to rubbing. *Differential diagnosis*: listeriosis (**459**) and meningitis (**465**).

461
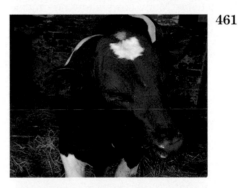

Facial nerve paralysis

In **462** the ear, upper eyelid and muzzle are drooping. In this bull the cause was unknown, but possible aetiology includes trauma, middle ear disease, listeriosis and other brain infections. *Differential diagnosis*: includes botulism (**687**), rabies (**478**) and listeriosis (**459**).

462
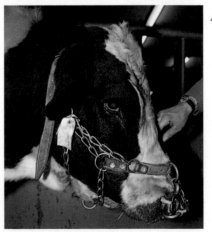

Brain abscess

The Ayrshire cow in **463** looks apprehensive, holds her head to one side and is unable to stand on her front legs. An abscess (A) was seen in the base of the brain on postmortem (**464**). A common location for such abscesses is the pituitary fossa.

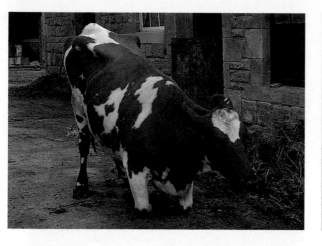

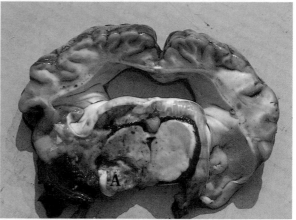

Meningitis

Meningitis produces a range of clinical signs. The calf in **465** is pushing its head against the wall, its pupils are dilated and it is frothing at the mouth. Some calves (**466**) are recumbent and dull, with drooping ears and eyelids, giving the appearance of an intense headache. Adult cows may also be affected.

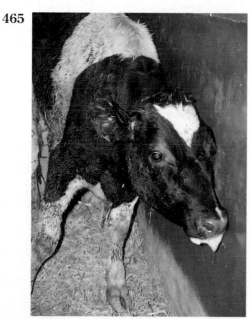

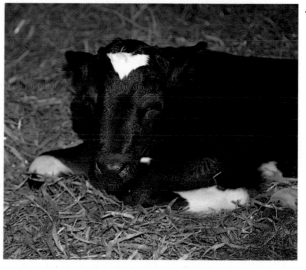

The calf in **466** exhibited a hypopyon (**467**) which rapidly resolved following treatment. A more extreme case developed extensor spasm (**468**) and opisthotonos (**469**), but recovered. Adult cattle can be affected. A range of organisms may be involved including *Strep-* *tococci* (**470** shows a congested brain at postmortem), *Haemophilus*, *Pasteurella* and *Listeria*. *Differential diagnosis*: rabies (**478–481**), brain abscess (**463**), acute lead poisoning (**726**) and infectious thromboembolic meningoencephalitis (**471**).

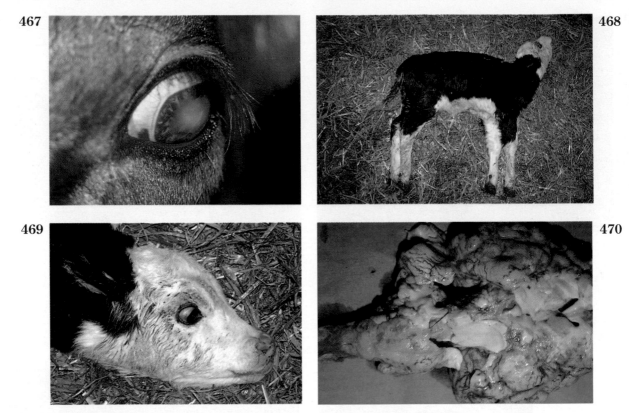

Infectious thromboembolic meningoencephalitis (TEME, ITEME) or infectious septic thrombomeningoencephalomyelitis (ISTEM, ISTMEM)

Infectious thromboembolic meningoencephalitis is seen primarily in feedlot cattle and is caused by *Haemophilus somnus*. The correct terminology is disputed. This multisystemic condition is sudden in onset, occurring initially with marked pyrexia. Affected animals are dull and severely depressed, as in the Charolais bull in **471**. Note the salivation, drooping ears and eyelids. Recumbency and death may follow within a

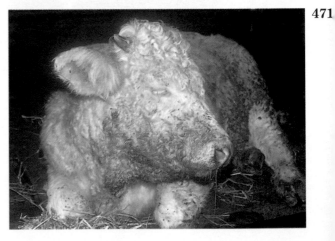

few hours. Blindness from retinal haemorrhages (**472**) and oedema are early features. Marked cerebral oedema, congestion and haemorrhage are seen in a ventral view of the brain (**473**) at postmortem, with congestion of the grey matter, cerebral haemorrhages (in the lateral ventricles), meningitis and discoloured cerebrospinal fluid (CSF) as in the transverse section (**474**). *H. somnus* alone can cause a suppurative bronchopneumonia (**475**) with severe cranioventral changes evident, or it may be involved in shipping fever or pasteurellosis (**231**).

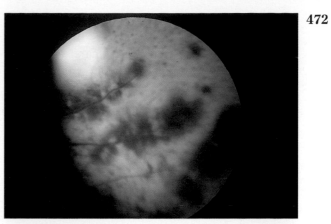

472

73

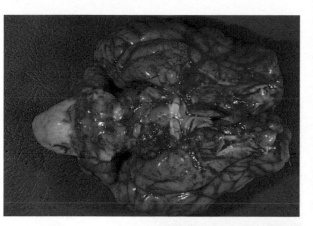

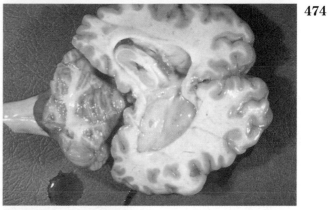

474

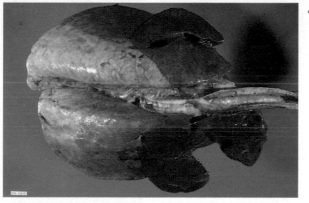

475

Coenurus cerebralis ('gid')

Coenurus cerebralis is the intermediate stage of the canine tapeworm, *Taenia multiceps*. It occasionally encysts in cattle brains, producing a slow, progressive nervous disease. Starting with blindness, head pushing and aimless wandering, affected animals eventually become recumbent over a period of 1–4 months. The cyst often lies immediately beneath the frontal bone, from where it can be removed from the external surface of the cerebral hemispheres. This animal made a full recovery (**476**).

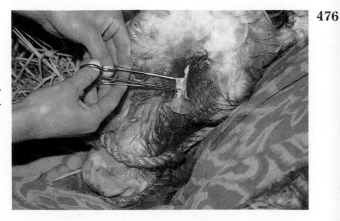

476

Viral infections

Rabies

477

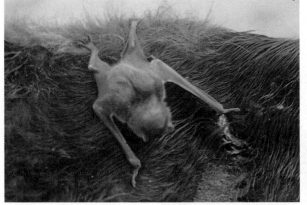

478

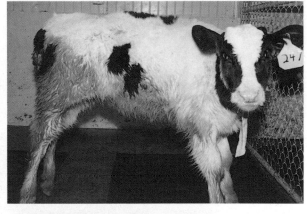

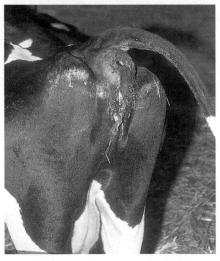

479

Rabies is a rhabdoviral infection that produces a fatal encephalomyelitis. Dogs, cats and wild carnivores are primarily affected, but the disease can occur in all warm-blooded animals, including cattle and man. Carrier animals transmit infective saliva to cattle by biting, e.g., the vampire bat shown feeding from a cow in Brazil in **477**, was later found to harbour the rabies virus. The virus then passes to the brain via peripheral nerves, hence the variation in incubation period depending on the site of injury. Initially seen simply as a change in behaviour, early cases progress to show salivation, apprehension, and knuckling of the hind fetlocks, as in the Friesian calf in **478**. Some cattle show marked tenesmus (**479**). This may lead directly to paralysis and death, although the more classic 'furious' form of rabies, with characteristic bellowing (**480**), aggression and salivation (**481**), can sometimes also occur in cattle. Countries free of rabies maintain strict quarantine measures for dogs and cats entering from abroad. Many other countries have active eradication campaigns and a compulsory vaccination policy for certain domestic species. *Differential diagnosis*: bacterial meningitis (**465**), brain abscess (**463**), listeriosis (**459**), botulism (**688**), Aujeszky's disease (**482**) and nervous ketosis (**457**).

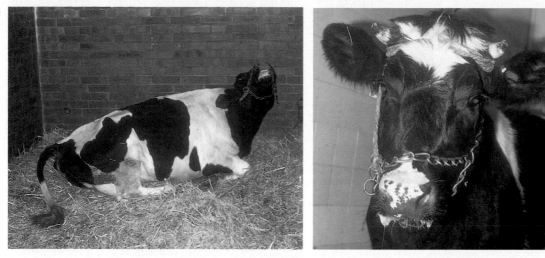

Aujeszky's disease (pseudorabies, 'mad itch')

Although Aujeszky's disease is primarily a herpes virus infection of pigs, other species, including cattle, can develop a meningoencephalitis that is usually fatal within 48 hours. Apprehension, licking, trembling and salivation (**482**) are early signs, typically followed by an intense pruritus. The grossly swollen eyelids in **482** are the result of intense rubbing to relieve the pruritus.

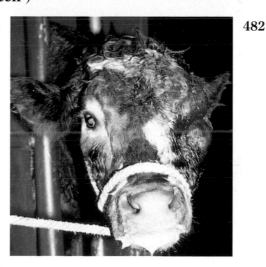

Bovine spongiform encephalopathy (BSE)

Cows (generally of dairy breeds) that are between three and six years old are primarily affected by bovine spongiform encephalopathy. Occasional cases occur in bulls. Clinical signs include weight loss (**483**), an unsteady, stiff-legged gait, especially in the hind legs, and behavioural changes such as teeth grinding, muscle twitching, nervousness and aggression. Severe posterior ataxia and, eventually, recumbency develop after a period of days to months. The change in gait is difficult to visualise in a photograph. The Friesian cow in **484** shows an arched back and excessive straightness of the hind legs as she turns to her left. She was difficult (almost dangerous) to handle. Typical microscopic spongiform changes were seen in the brain at postmortem.

First seen in 1986, BSE is largely confined to the UK, Eire and Switzerland at the present time. The precise cause is unknown, but ingestion of a scrapie-like agent in feedstuffs has been strongly implicated. Susceptibility to infection is possibly inherited. The disease is now notifiable in Britain. *Differential diagnosis:* rabies (**477–481**), Aujeszky's disease (**482**), meningitis (**465–470**), brain abscess (**463–464**) and hypomagnesaemia (**453–454**).

483

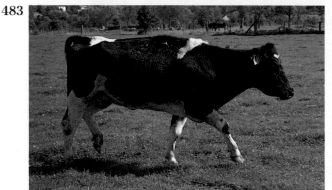

484

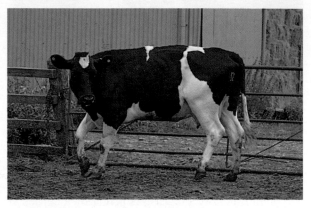

Pruritis–pyrexia–haemorrhagica (PPH)

In PPH, raised plaques of skin on the head (**485**), neck, tail and udder resemble ringworm (**88 & 89**), but are intensely pruritic. More severe cases are pyrexic, anorexic and pass blood from the mouth, nose and rectum. The cause is unknown, but a fungal toxin, producing white, necrotic renal foci, and sweet vernal grass have both been implicated. *Differential diagnosis*: Aujeszky's disease (**482**), mange (**77**), and ringworm (**88**).

485

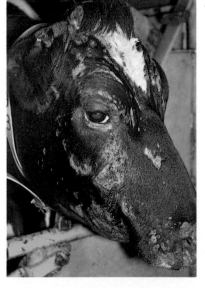

Salt-craving pica

Prolonged, deficient diets lead to an intense craving for salt. Affected animals will often lick and bite any object (pica), and may avidly attack salt blocks (**486**). Milk production, food intake, growth and fertility may be depressed.

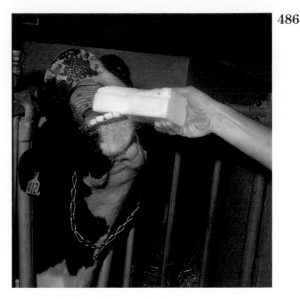

Lightning stroke

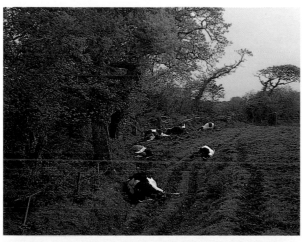

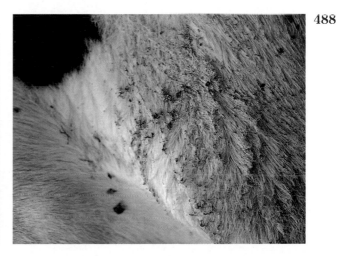

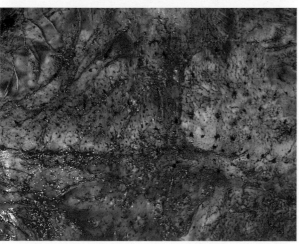

Animals that have been struck by lightning are typically found beside a hedge, a wire fence (**487**), or under a tree. The tree may show evidence of lightening damage. Trees that have shallow-spreading root systems are particularly dangerous, especially if the ground is damp or has underground drains. Dead animals may be found with fresh food in the mouth and scorch marks of burned hair on the coat, especially on the legs (**488**). Removal of the hide reveals extensive bleeding due to rupture of the subcutaneous blood vessels (**489**). Mildly affected animals may recover after a variable period of time. *Differential diagnosis* (of sudden death): hypomagnesaemia (**453**), bloat (**180**), pulmonary thromboembolism (**251–254**), cardiac failure (see Chapter 6), anthrax (**682**).

Electrocution

Electrocution is quite commonly seen in cattle, partly owing to an inherent susceptibility, and partly because they are more often exposed in milking parlours (**490**). Clinical signs vary from being stunned, with resulting nasal, oral and ocular bleeding, to death (as in the cows in **490**), also with profuse bleeding. Death is due to ventricular fibrillation and respiratory arrest. Exposure to lower levels of high amperage electric current produces a variety of nervous and behavioural changes, depending on the voltage intensity.

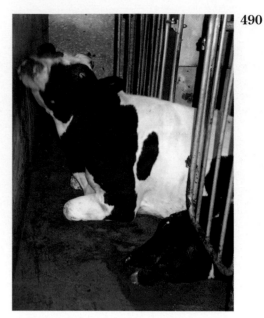

490

10 Urinogenital disorders

Urinary tract
Introduction

The main infectious and bacterial diseases of the bovine urinary tract are pyelonephritis and leptospirosis. Urolithiasis is a multifactorial urinary problem resulting from metabolic and nutritional disorders. Finally, amyloidosis, although an uncommon sporadic disease of adult cattle, requires differentiation from pyelonephritis.

Conditions with secondary renal pathology include pruritus–pyrexia–haemorrhagica (PPH) (**485**), oak (acorn) poisoning (**703** & **704**), renal infarction secondary to caudal vena caval thrombosis (**255**), and babesiosis (redwater, **655**).

Pyelonephritis

491
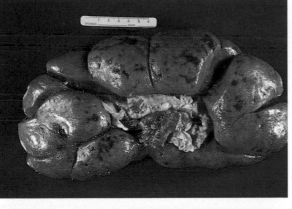

492
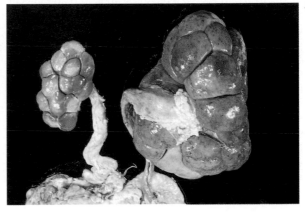

493
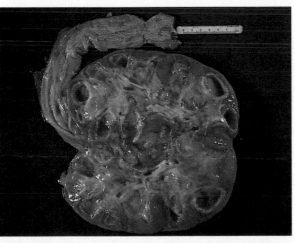

A mature cow with uraemia shows superficial, dark areas of infected thrombi in an enlarged kidney (**491**) from which *Corynebacterium renale* was cultured. In **492** and **493** severe chronic pyelonephritis is illustrated. In **492** the left kidney is contracted and pale, and the right kidney is enlarged and appears granular. Both ureters, particularly the left, are thickened as they contain pus and cellular debris (pyoureter). In **493**, the sectioned kidney of an active case (in a five-year-old Charolais cow) shows multiple caseous and purulent centres, primarily in the medulla. The numerous blood-filled cavities are septic foci. The third example of pyelonephritis (**494**) shows renal calculi in the calyces, further calculi within the lumen of a thickened ureter, and multiple petechiae (A) on the mucosa of the bladder wall.

Pyelonephritis is usually an infection that ascends from the vagina and vulva. Caused by *Corynebacterium renale*, it may result from contact with infected urine or from a genital tract infection. Affected cows are pyrexic, lose weight, and may develop a dry, brownish discolouration of the coat.

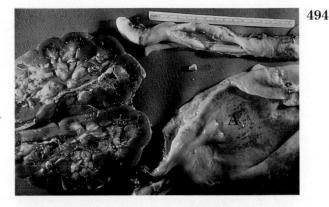

Leptospirosis

The main effects of *Leptospira interrogans* serovar. *pomona* or *hardjo* infection are abortion (see **575** for a foetus from a possible leptospiral abortion) and loss of milk production in adult cattle. When *pomona* only is involved, an acute septicaemia, with haemoglobinuria, jaundice, anaemia and possible death, is seen in calves. Dark swollen kidneys (**495**) are usually indicative of a haemolytic crisis. Recovered cattle show little more than ill-defined, greyish, cortical spots, indicative of a focal interstitial nephritis. The spirochaete may be seen under dark field microscopy of urine, but confirmation of diagnosis otherwise depends on serology or histopathology. *Differential diagnosis:* babesiosis (**655–660**), anaplasmosis (**661–664**), rape and kale poisoning (**707**), post-parturient haemoglobinuria, and bacil-

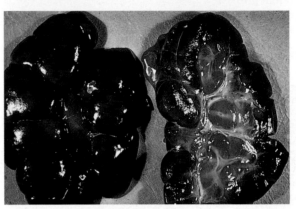
495

lary haemoglobinuria (**213**). Note the completely different appearances of the kidney in pyelonephritis (**491–493**) and amyloidosis (**504**).

Urolithiasis

Urolithiasis has a multifactorial aetiology including a relatively reduced fluid intake, mineral imbalance, high concentrate intake and castration. The condition begins with microcalculus formation in the kidneys, and clinical problems arise when the calculi grow to a sufficient size to obstruct the urethra.

Although preputial crystals (often struvite, i.e., magnesium–ammonium–phosphate hexahydrate) appear in many calves (**496**), relatively few will develop signs of obstruction, which tends to occur in or just

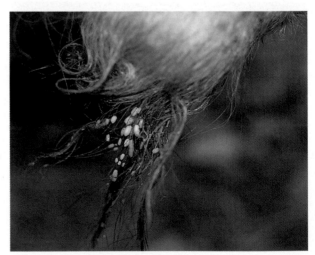
496

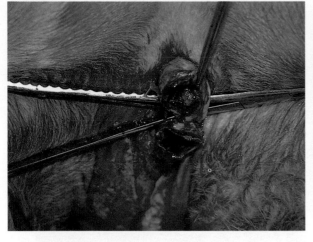

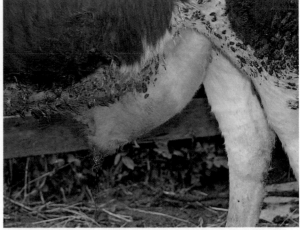

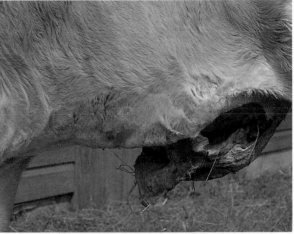

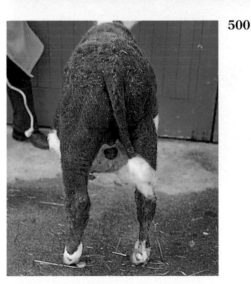

proximal to the sigmoid flexure, or in the distal portion of the penis. An intraoperative view (**497**) of the perineal region shows the dilated urethra proximal to the sigmoid flexure and the obstructing calculus. If complete urethral obstruction persists, either bladder or, more commonly, urethral rupture occurs. The Hereford steer in **498** has a large subcutaneous swelling containing urine as a result of urethral rupture in the sigmoid region. The swelling extends forwards from the sigmoid to the preputial orifice, which is discoloured and shows dry preputial hairs covered with crystals. Sometimes the swelling is unusually discretely localised to the peripreputial area. In contrast, in the severe and advanced case in **499**, the Friesian steer had such severe swelling that ischaemic necrosis has caused an extensive skin slough overlying the penis. *Differential diagnosis*: in a mature bull this includes penile haematoma (**514**) or abscess formation, or, in a younger animal, urethral rupture due to faulty application of a bloodless castrator (Burdizzo) some days previously (see p.161).

In another Hereford steer (**500**) it is the bladder rather than the urethra that has ruptured as a result of urethral obstruction, and urine has gathered in the ventral abdominal cavity, causing a progressive swelling and distension of the flanks. *Differential diagnosis*: for ventral abdominal swelling this includes ascites (**207**), intestinal obstruction (**204**), and generalised peritonitis with massive exudation (**206**).

Postmortem examination of a six-year-old Shorthorn bull that died as a result of severe uraemia following bladder rupture and uroperitoneum, reveals a congested and haemorrhagic bladder mucosa (**501**). Numerous calculi (2–7mm diameter) and fibrin are seen on the mucosal surface. In **502** the peritoneum is diffusely inflamed, but the changes are less severe than those following septic reticuloperitonitis (**205 & 206**). Urolithiasis is frequently seen in cases of severe pyelonephritis (**494**). *Differential diagnosis:* includes cystitis (**505**), urethral obstruction (**497–500**), severe balanoposthitis (**518–520**) and severe preputial frostbite.

501
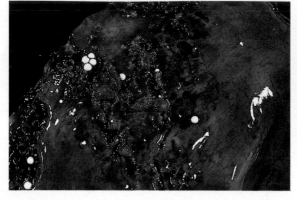

502
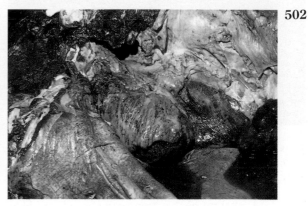

Amyloidosis

The marked presternal oedema in the three-year-old Limousin bull in **503** was caused by severe bilateral amyloidosis, which is characterised by polyuria and massive proteinuria leading to pronounced hypoproteinaemia.

Secondary amyloidosis is associated with chronic suppurative conditions. The bull's kidney in **504** is markedly enlarged, pale, waxy and granular in comparison with the normal kidney above. This degree of enlargement should be detectable on rectal palpation.

503
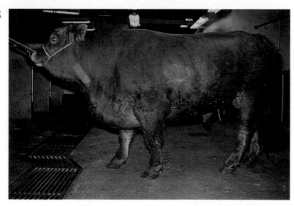

504
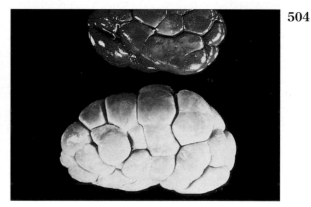

Cystitis

The six-month-old heifer in **505** passed urine frequently and in small amounts. The perineal region had a foul odour of stale urine and shows excoriation as a result of urine dribbling. The tail is slightly elevated (urinary tenesmus).

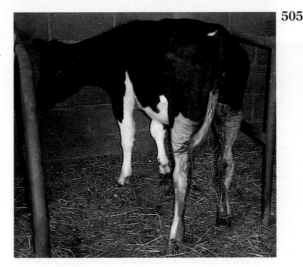

505

Male genitalia

Introduction

The anatomical separation of parts of the male genital tract, and their common development with parts of the urinary tract, makes integration of this section difficult. The section starts with congenital conditions, and continues with abnormalities affecting the penis, prepuce, scrotum, and, finally, the epididymis and seminal vesicles. Some congenital anomalies (e.g., persistent frenulum, cryptorchidism and testicular hypoplasia) may not become apparent until breeding age (1–2 years old).

Congenital male genital abnormalities

Pseudohermaphrodite

In the one-year-old Africander bull in **506** the preputial opening and galea glandis are shown at A. The penis is situated at the ischium and, although the scrotum is absent, the testes are in the inguinal region. The condition is rare. The animal may be mistaken for female at birth owing to the origin of the urinary flow. The umbilicus usually has a skin fold reminiscent of the prepuce.

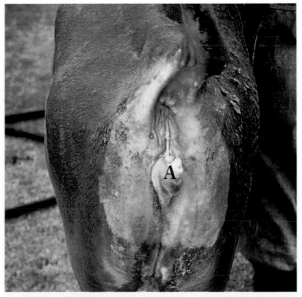

506

Persistent frenulum

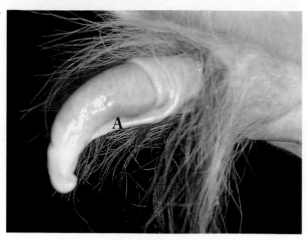

In **507** the penile body remains attached to the prepuce by a fine, longitudinal band(A). Persistent penile frenulum causing penile deviation is a congenital anomaly, but signs, such as ventral penile deviation or a failure of complete protrusion, are usually first seen at attempted intromission. The cause is incomplete separation of the penis and prepuce along the ventral raphé during the first year. In some breeds it is inherited, and surgically corrected bulls should not be used to sire replacement animals.

Testicular hypoplasia with cryptorchidism

The left testicle is descended and of normal size in the Friesian calf in **508**. The right testicle, which is small and incompletely descended, is in the scrotal neck.

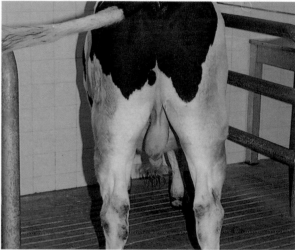

508

Cryptorchidism

509

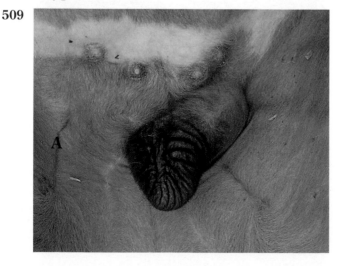

Bovine cryptorchidism, which is rare, is possibly associated with the polled character. In the four-week old Hereford cross calf in **509**, the normal right testicle is in the scrotal sac, but the left testicle is in an inguinal position (A). The misplaced gonad has deviated from the normal course of descent and may be termed an 'ectopic testicle'.

Penile conditions

Fibropapilloma

The two-year-old Friesian bull in **510** has several highly vascular, ulcerated masses attached to the glans penis. Caudal to the large mass is a smaller, more sessile fibropapilloma. These are typical sites for such multiple, proliferating masses, which are in-fectious, of viral origin, and relatively common in groups of young bulls confined in a small area. Four months later the mass had largely spontaneously disappeared (**511**), and the bull could be used for natural service.

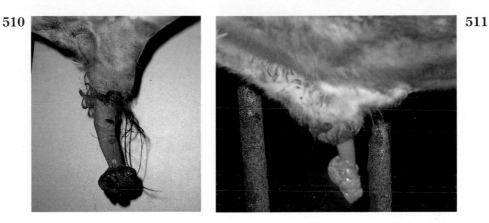

510   511

Spiral deviation of penis ('corkscrew penis')

Spiral or corkscrew is the most common form of pe-nile deviation. It is a normal occurrence at ejaculation, but premature corkscrewing may be severe enough to prevent intromission. The first case, a two-year-old Charolais, shows a 90⁰ ventral curvature (**512**). The second case (**513**) clearly illustrates the spiralling effect, and the difficulty of intromission. In some bulls, an ulcer on the glans penis indicates abrasion from repeated perineal contact. Spiral deviation is due to slipping of the dorsal apical ligament of the penis and may occur intermittently.

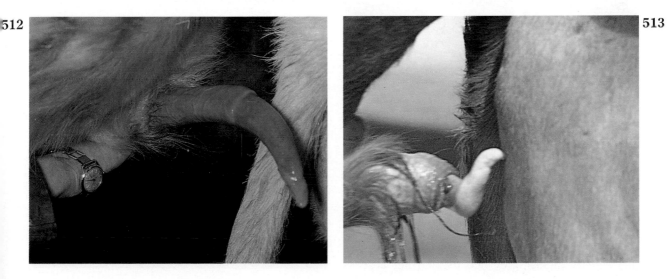

512   513

Penile and parapenile haematoma ('fracture of penis', 'broken penis')

A discrete swelling is seen in the Hereford bull in **514**, which also had a secondary prolapse of the penis. The tunica albuginea is ruptured, producing a prescrotal haematoma and oedema. This rupture involves the corpus cavernosum penis (CCP) and is almost always through the dorsal wall of the tunica, just distal to the sigmoid flexure. The extent of the ruptured CCP is evident in the postmortem specimen of an affected penis (**515**). Rupture occurs at ejaculation, or, less commonly, at intromission when the fully engorged penis is suddenly bent beyond its physiological limits, for example, when the cow or heifer suddenly moves.

514

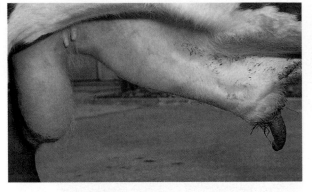

515

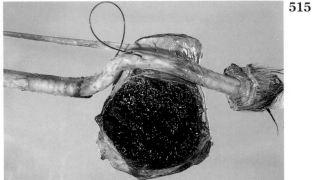

Preputial conditions

Prolapsed prepuce (preputial eversion)

516

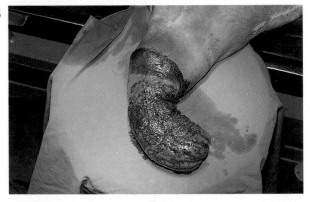

Preputial prolapse occurs as a breed characteristic in *Bos indicus*, e.g., Brahman and Santa Gertrudis, and in polled breeds. A partial preputial prolapse of comparatively recent onset is shown in a six-year-old Brahman from South Africa (**516**). The mucosa has a granular appearance, with areas of superficial haemorrhage. More severe cases are very prone to secondary trauma and oedema.

Preputial and penile abscess

In the five-year-old Hereford bull in **517**, the penis has been manually prolapsed. The hand holds the prepuce and penis just caudal to the point of attachment of the preputial mucosa (internal lamina) to the body of the penis, shown as a transverse fold. Pus oozes from a mucosal tear incurred when the penis was extended. Deep-red erectile tissue is evident in the defect. Below the wound, the mucosa is smooth and slightly pinkish-grey due to a further abscess pocket.

517

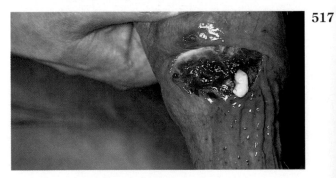

Posthitis and balanoposthitis

Posthitis is an inflammation of the prepuce. The post-mortem specimen of an eight-year-old Santa Gertrudis in **518** shows severe necrosis of the preputial mucosa both at the skin–mucosa margin, and more caudally.

Balanoposthitis is an inflammation of both the prepuce and the penis. The Jersey bull in **519** shows chronic fibrotic changes that involved both penile and preputial mucosae, causing adhesions. In the Hereford bull in **520**, the penis is partially extruded to illustrate the marked congestion and inflammatory reaction on the preputial mucosa. The preputial orifice (A) is swollen as a result of the posthitis. The paler penis has several discrete papules. Some cases of balanoposthitis are due to genital IBR infection (**227**), while others are of traumatic origin.

518   **519**   **520**

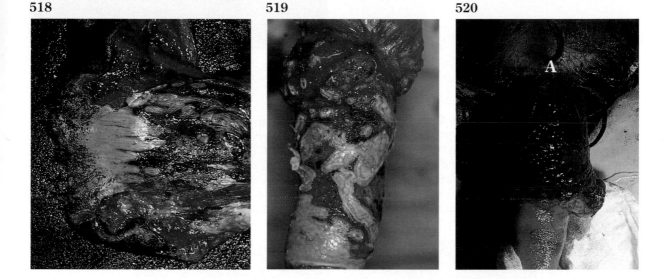

Scrotal conditions

Inguinal hernia

There is a soft, reducible swelling in the inguinal region overlying the two rudimentary teats in this Sussex bull from Zimbabwe (**521**). Neither the scrotal neck nor the body is enlarged, showing that only the inguinal canal is involved. An inguinal hernia may contain omentum, or both omentum and small intestinal loops. Cattle have a genetic predisposition to inguinal hernia, inheritance being recessive. Affected bulls should not be used to sire replacement stock. In over-conditioned animals it can be difficult to differentiate fat deposits from a hernia.

521

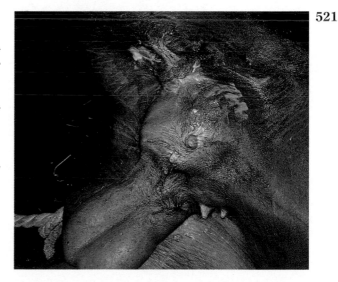

Scrotal hernia

In 522 a six-year-old Hereford bull shows an obvious swelling in the left side of the scrotal neck. It was soft, painless and partially reducible. This scrotal hernia resulted in the production of very poor quality semen. The hernia had been acquired as a result of traumatic injury, and was not congenital. Scrotal hernia is rare in cattle.

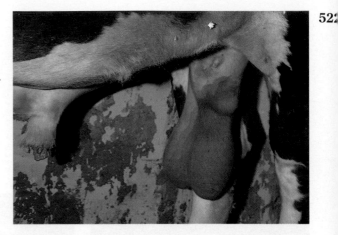

Orchitis

In **523** the scrotum of a four-year-old Simmental bull shows enlargement of the right testis, which is more dependent than the left. Note that the scrotal neck is not swollen. The testis was painful and sensitive to touch. The aetiology of this unilateral orchitis was probably traumatic, although various pathogens, including *Brucella abortus, Mycobacterium tuberculosis* and *Actinomyces pyogenes*, have been isolated. In the acute *Brucella* orchitis illustrated in **524**, the inflammatory reaction in the tunics and epididymis caused a severe periorchitis (pale areas (A)), with early testicular necrosis as a result of testicular enlargement, and compression by the tunica albuginea. Ventrally, oedematous fluid lies subcutaneously (B).

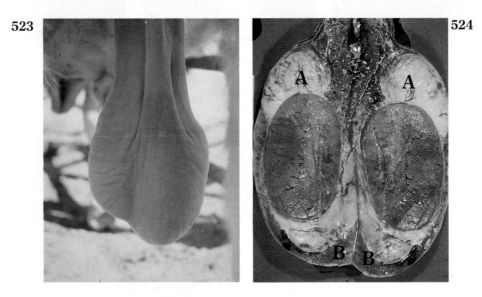

523

524

Scirrhous cord

The scrotum is very swollen in the four-month-old Friesian calf in **525**. A dried blood clot lies over the ventral scrotal incision (castration). Exploration revealed an enlarged stump of the spermatic cord, which resulted from infection acquired at surgery. Such wounds predispose calves to tetanus.

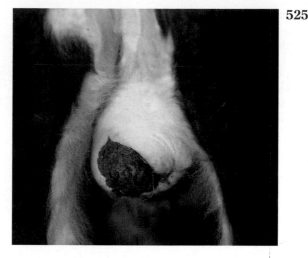

Scrotal necrosis and gangrene

The Friesian calf in **526** has an irregular necrotic line at the scrotal neck, separating gangrenous from normal tissue. The reaction is a result of faulty application of a bloodless castrator (Burdizzo). A continuous, crushed line encircles the scrotal neck, cutting off the blood supply to the lower skin. The same effect is obtained when a rubber castration ring is placed around the scrotal neck, and all tissue distal to the ring undergoes atrophy. When this is done relatively late on, i.e., after one week old, the reaction is much more severe. In the Friesian in **527** the ring was applied at two months. Note the considerable swelling proximal to the ring, compared with the shrivelled, dark, necrotic, distal portion.

If a bloodless castrator is applied too high, the urethra may be accidentally crushed, leading to urethral rupture, and a ventral, subcutaneous accumulation of urine similar to that following calculus obstruction (**499**). Many countries have legal (statutory) limits on the age at which Burdizzo and rubber ring castration may be carried out.

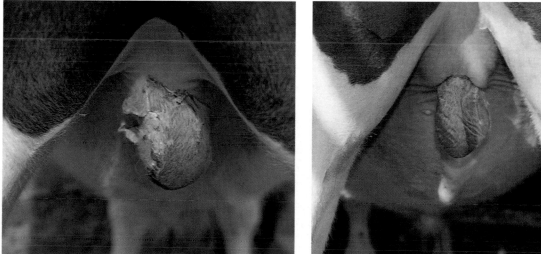

Scrotal frostbite

Moderate frostbite affected the bottom of the scrotum of a two-year-old Simmental (**528**) following exposure to a temperature of −30°C in Saskatchewan, Canada, 2–8 weeks previously. The semen quality was poor (<10% live cells). Most cases return to normal semen quality within 2–3 months.

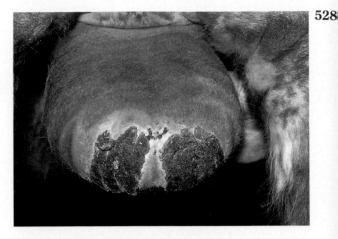

Seminal vesiculitis

Although the right seminal vesicle of the bull in **529** is normal and the ampulla has its lumen exposed, the left ampulla is absent and the left seminal vesicle shows cystic, haemorrhagic and mild inflammatory changes. Seminal vesiculitis causes a purulent, preputial discharge after service, or pus may be seen in semen collected for artificial insemination (AI). Common organisms include *Actinomyces pyogenes*, *Brucella* and *Escherichia coli*. Young bulls are predominantly involved. Seminal vesiculitis is readily diagnosed by rectal palpation. Lack of symmetry, firmness and pain are the significant findings.

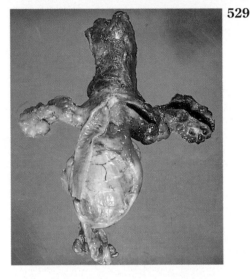

Female genitalia

Introduction

Maintenance of optimum fertility is of major economic importance in both beef and dairy herds. A high lifetime output of milk and calves can only be attained if cows breed regularly, and considerable effort is expended on veterinary fertility examinations, health control, disease prevention and optimising nutrition to achieve this. Much of this work cannot be adequately illustrated. For example, mineral and trace element deficiencies may affect fertility by reducing conception rates or interrupting ovarian cycles, but they cannot be demonstrated pictorially. Poor management techniques, particularly heat detection, which is very important, can often only be demonstrated by an analysis of records.

Diseases and disorders of the female genital tract are numerous. This chapter starts with a description of anatomical, congenital and developmental abnormalities, including cystic ovaries and neoplasia of the tract. The latter is comparatively rare. Dystocia is difficult to illustrate. Many conditions are diagnosed and corrected by intravaginal and intrauterine manipulation. Postpartum complications include vaginal wall rupture and haemorrhage, prolapse of parts of the genital tract (uterine prolapse is the most common) and metritis, endometritis and pyometra, all of which are sequelae of dystocia, which in turn is commonly the result of poor bull selection. There is often a conflict of interest between the use of a large breed bull to produce valuable offspring and a small breed to facilitate easy parturition. Not all pregnancies reach term and the final section of the chapter illustrates some causes of abortion and premature calving.

Congenital abnormalities

Intersexuality and freemartinism result from placental fusion in early pregnancy. Segmental aplasia of the müllerian duct system is inherited and leads to a range of abnormalities including white heifer disease (imperforate hymen). Ovarian agenesis, ovarian hypoplasia and fallopian tube aplasia have all been reported, but they are rare and, therefore, are not illustrated.

Freemartinism

530

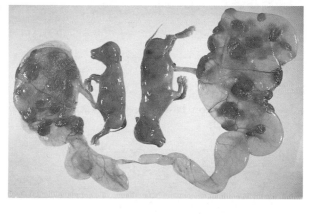

531

532

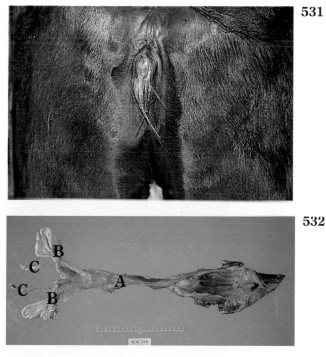

In cattle, over 90% of twin calves have fused placentae, with a common blood supply. **530** shows how small the point of fusion may be. The heifer calf starts its development as a female, but, owing to the interchange of embryonic cells and hormones between the thirtieth and fortieth days of pregnancy (i.e., before the stage of sexual dimorphism), many develop male characteristics. The freemartin is probably masculinised by the secretion from its own gonads. The Friesian heifer in **531** has an enlarged clitoris, and excess hair is growing as a tuft from the ventral vulval commissure. On rectal examination, no internal genitalia could be palpated beyond the cervix. Varying degrees of hypoplasia and masculinisation may be seen. **532** demonstrates hypoplasia of the anterior vagina (A), an absence of the cervix, vestigial ovaries (B) and testes (C) that are joined to the immature uterine horns by ducts.

Segmental uterine aplasia ('white heifer disease', imperforate hymen)

Segmental uterine aplasia is a developmental defect of the müllerian duct system, in which ovarian development allows normal oestrus behaviour, but the hymen is often persistent. Pregnancy may occur in mild cases, with the persistent hymen sometimes leading to dystocia. In the advanced case shown in **533**, the right uterine horn is aplastic, the residual portion (A) being dilated with cyclical fluid. This could be classified as uterus unicornis. The condition is due to a sex-linked recessive gene, but, despite its popular name of white heifer disease, it is not always related to coat colour.

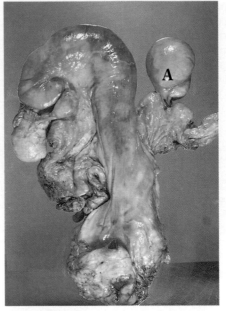

533

Double cervix (double os uteri externum)

Only the external cervical os is duplicated in this second example of a müllerian duct defect (**534**). An endoscopic view (**535**) illustrates placental membranes, visible through the left (upper dark) os. This inherited condition leads to surprisingly few incidents of dystocia.

534

535

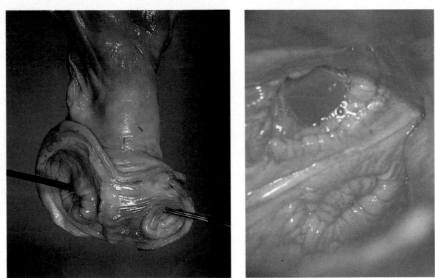

Cystic ovaries

Ovarian cysts arise from a failure of ovulation. The anovulatory follicle increases in size to produce a fluid-filled structure greater than 2.5cm in diameter, and normal ovarian cycles are usually interrupted. Occasionally, cysts develop during pregnancy. Stress, deficiencies, feeding for high milk yields and heredity are among the suggested causes. Although classically subdivided into luteal and follicular cysts, there is probably a degree of interchange between the two states. Many cysts resolve spontaneously, whilst others require treatment.

Luteal cyst

In **536** a single, large, spherical, thick-walled cyst is present in the left ovary. Luteal cysts secrete progesterone and may lead to prolonged anoestrus. The right ovary contains an incised cystic corpus luteum, a structure which does not impede normal cyclical behaviour.

536

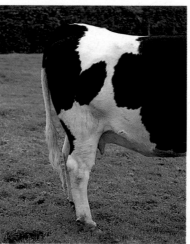

Follicular cyst

In **537** the right ovary contains a large, thin-walled follicular cyst. Such cysts are invariably oestrogenic and lead to irregular or prolonged oestrus periods. Multilocular follicular cysts frequently occur. A corpus luteum, 5–7 days old, is present in the left ovary, suggesting that normal cyclicity can continue in the non-affected ovary. Cows with unresolved follicular cysts may develop a raised tail head as a result of relaxation of the pelvic ligaments (**538**), and characteristically male behavioural changes, such as deep bellowing and pawing the ground.

537

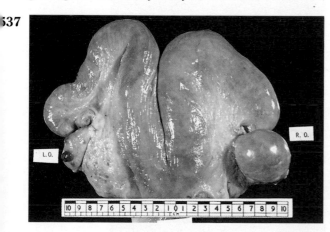

538

Bursal adhesions and hydrosalpinx

The bursa in **539** is tightly adherent to a large cyst in the right ovary, the oviduct (A) of which is distended with fluid (hydrosalpinx). The small visible portion (B) of the left oviduct is normal and the left ovary contains a 3–5-day-old corpus luteum (C). Bursal adhesions can result from rough handling of the ovary in, for example, manual rupture of ovarian cysts and enucleation of corpora lutea.

Hydrosalpinx is more pronounced in the oviduct of **540**, which is grossly distended with fluid (A) following a loss of patency. A small segment of normal duct (B) is visible on the bursa, as well as a 6–8-day-old corpus luteum on the ovary (C). The aetiology may involve inflammation arising from an ascending uterine infection or be traumatic, for example, following manual ovarian manipulation.

539 **540**

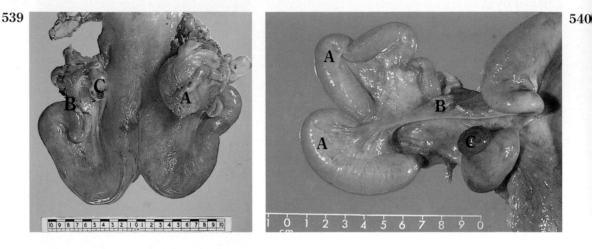

Female genital tract tumours

Granulosa cell tumours are by far the most common ovarian neoplasms, but fibromas, sarcomas and carcinomas have been reported. Uterine fibromyomas, leiomyomas and lymphosarcomas are rare, whilst fibropapillomas (polyps) of the vagina and cervix are not uncommon.

Ovarian granulosa cell tumour

A large cystic neoplasm is seen in the right ovary in **541**. Initially oestrogen-secreting, such tumours cause nymphomania. Advanced cases undergo luteinisation, leading to anoestrus or even masculinisation. The incised uterine horn shows endometrial hyperplasia and mucometra.

541

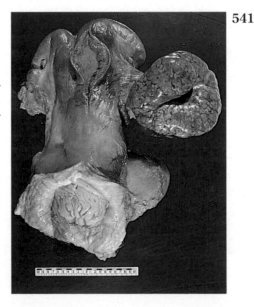

Uterine fibromyoma

Seen as a smooth mass involving much of the uterine wall (**542**), this type of tumour does not necessarily interrupt pregnancy. Tumours of the uterus and cervix are rare in cattle.

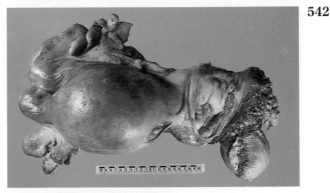

Hydrops allantois (hydrops amnii)

In hydrops allantois (hydrallantois) the lower abdomen is grossly distended bilaterally as a result of excess fluid accumulating in the uterus, usually in the allantoic sac (**543**). The condition develops progressively in the seventh to ninth months of pregnancy, causing death of the foetus, and may result in the rupture of the prepubic tendon (**121**). Fluid volumes of up to 300 litres have been recorded (normal volume is 8–10 litres). Shock, dystocia and retained placenta are common complications, which frequently are fatal.

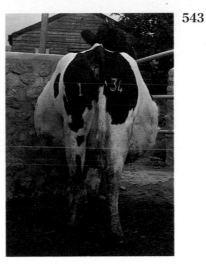

Dystocia

Dystocia in cattle may be due to twins, foetal postural defects, foetal monstrosities (e.g., anasarca, **548**, and schistosomus reflexus, **8**), maternal problems (e.g., uterine torsion), and disproportion between foetal and maternal size. The latter is the most common cause, especially in heifers, and typically results from small undersized heifers, or from inappropriate bull selection leading to an oversized foetus, or from the restriction of available space in the pelvic birth canal by maternal overfeeding. The conditions illustrated in this section are chosen as examples. The list is by no means comprehensive.

Head only presentation

The case in **544** is not a long-standing dystocia, as the head is moist and of normal size. The shoulders will be at the pelvic inlet, the forelimbs in the uterus.

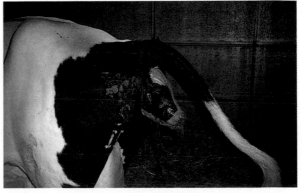

Head and one leg presentation

In **545** a more long-standing case of dystocia (leg back) is illustrated. The head and tongue are swollen and oedematous and the head is dry. The enlarged and oedematous vulval lips may persist for 24–48 hours after parturition.

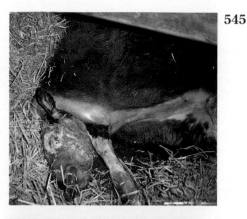

545

Posterior presentation, with foetal dorsoventral rotation

Initial observation of the calf's feet and fetlocks in **546** might suggest a case of anterior presentation, with lateral deviation of the head (head back). Closer inspection shows the hocks at the vulva, but the point of the hock is ventral. Rotation facilitated delivery of a live calf.

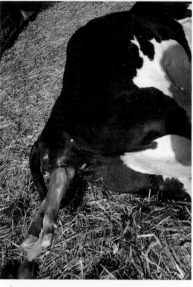

546

Breech presentation (hip flexion)

In **547** only the tail is visible and there is no vulval enlargement. Since insufficient foetal mass can enter the birth canal to stimulate abdominal contractions, many breech presentations pass unrecognised for several hours, or even days, and the calf is stillborn.

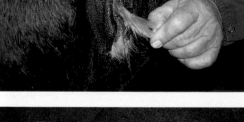

547

Anasarca

Note the subcutaneous oedema over the head, chest and abdomen in the anasarca calf in **548**. A neglected case, it led to maternal death from uterine rupture Foetal anasarca in Ayrshires is hereditary. Other foetal monstrosities leading to dystocia include arthrogryposis (**12**), schistosomus reflexus (**8**), perosomus elumbus and ascites.

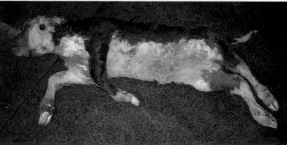

548

Uterine torsion

The anterior vagina can be seen to be rotated clockwise (**549**). About 75% of cases involve an anticlockwise torsion of 90–360°. Torsion develops at the very end of pregnancy, during late first-stage or early second-stage labour, and is usually associated with a large calf. A live calf was delivered from this cow, following correction of the torsion, but many are stillborn.

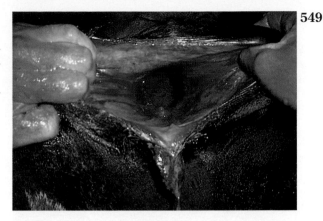

549

Post-partum complications

Normal, unassisted births result in few complications. However, after dystocia, particularly in cases of maternal disproportion involving considerable traction, complications are frequent. The most common is endometritis, which depresses subsequent fertility. Some of the more dramatic, but fortunately less frequent, complications illustrated here include vaginal wall rupture, uterine and other prolapses, rectovaginal fistula and septic vaginitis. A retained placenta can follow a normal parturition. Manual or endoscopic examinations of discharges from the cervix and anterior vagina play an important role in prebreeding examinations carried out as part of a herd fertility control programme. A range of discharges encountered has been illustrated with some gross uterine pathology.

Vaginal wall rupture and haemorrhage

Vaginal wall rupture with haemorrhage is a common complication, seen especially in overfat heifers with large calves, insufficient lubrication during traction, and excessively rapid traction that does not permit normal vaginal and vulval dilation. Preventive episiotomy is useful. Typically, the lateral vaginal wall tears approximately 10–20 cm from the vulval lips, at the level of the external urethral orifice. A large mass of pelvic fat may prolapse through the tear and protrude through the vulval lips (**550**). Rupture of the vaginal artery, a branch of the internal pudendal artery that is easily palpated in the lateral vaginal wall at the point of tearing, can result in severe and often fatal haemorrhage within an hour of parturition (**551**). Fortunately, the blood vessel was identified and ligated in this heifer, although she subsequently developed a severe perivaginitis and localised pelvic peritonitis.

550
551

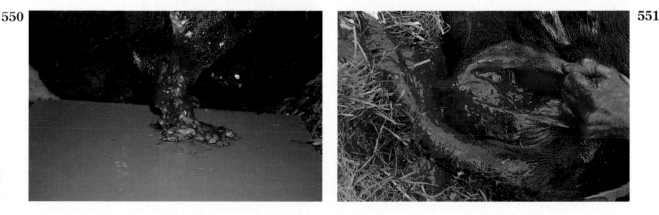

Rectovaginal fistula

Rectovaginal fistula is a complication of dystocia, resulting from an oversized foetus. In **552** (taken five days post-partum) the ventral anal mucosa is torn and there are extensive lacerations to the dorsal vaginal wall. The white material on the vaginal floor originates from intrauterine therapy. Three months later (**553**) the vaginal and anal lacerations had healed spontaneously, leaving a small, deformed area. Fertility is usually reduced, although this cow became pregnant in each of the next two years.

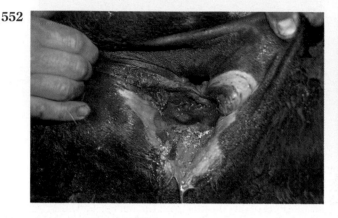

552

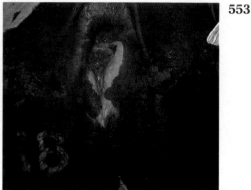

553

Septic vulvitis and vulvovaginitis

In **554** small, infected skin fissures are seen around the dorsal margin of the enlarged vulva, four days after the difficult delivery of an oversized calf. A length of placenta is seen in the ventral vulva. In severe cases of septic vulvitis the vulva is inflamed and oedematous, especially at the ventral commissure, and there is often a purulent haemorrhagic discharge from the vulva. A raised tail indicates discomfort. Vulval oedema and cellulitis are not always the result of trauma at parturition; the condition may also be the result of irritant faeces caused by acute diarrhoea.

Retained placenta

A retained placenta (**555**) is typically associated with factors that interfere with the third stage of labour, such as twins, prolonged parturition, excessive manual interference, abortion and premature calving, cows that are overfat or too thin, and certain mineral and trace element deficiencies, for example, selenium. In **555**, taken four days postpartum, the placenta is turning pink due to autolysis, and the udder is stained with a foul uterine discharge.

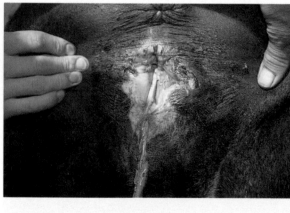

554

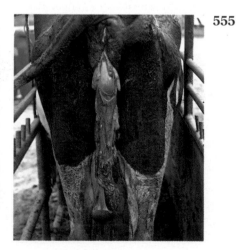

555

Vulval discharges, endometritis, metritis and pyometra

Vulval discharges may be associated with septic vulvovaginitis, a retained placenta, metritis and endometritis. Examination and treatment of endometritis is an important part of routine herd fertility control, especially in dairy herds. The type of discharge depends on the interval from calving to clinical examination, and on the degree of endometritis. Many discharges are normal and do not require treatment. Postoestral blood in clear mucus may be encountered (**556**). A plug of cervical mucus (**557**), which may be seen immediately prepartum or postpartum, is normal. Clear mucus containing pink streaks (**558**), and discoloured mucus containing red-brown material (**559**), or globules of yellow detritus (**560**), are also examples of lochia that would not normally be treated.

556

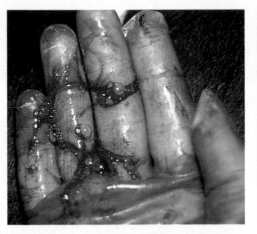

557

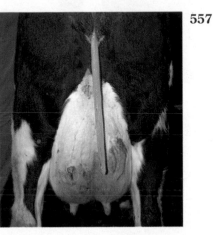

558

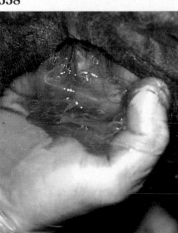

559

560

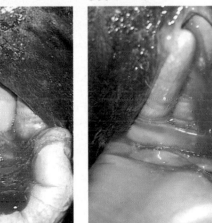

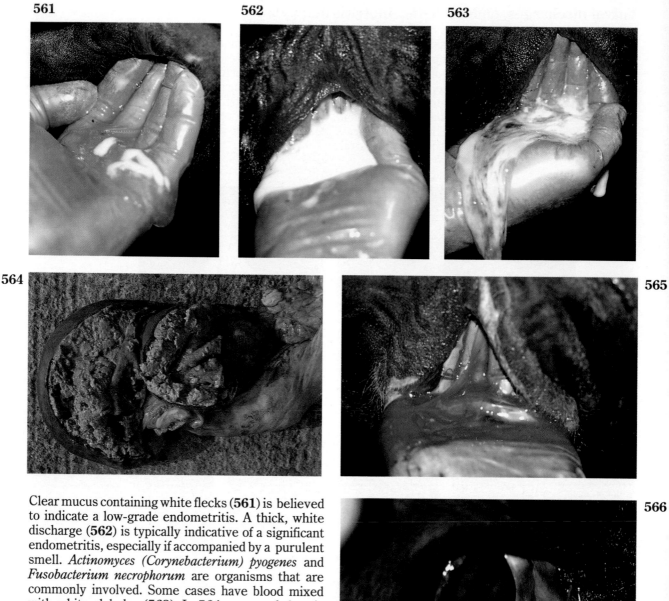

Clear mucus containing white flecks (**561**) is believed to indicate a low-grade endometritis. A thick, white discharge (**562**) is typically indicative of a significant endometritis, especially if accompanied by a purulent smell. *Actinomyces (Corynebacterium) pyogenes* and *Fusobacterium necrophorum* are organisms that are commonly involved. Some cases have blood mixed with white globules (**563**). In **564**, a case of chronic endometritis and pyometra, the incised uterine horns reveal a mass of caseous material. The enlarged uterus indicates a pyometra, which is an accumulation of uterine pus, with or without a vaginal discharge.

Metritis is indicated by a stinking, brown discharge (**565**), particularly when the discharge is fluid and not mucoid in consistency. Affected animals often show systemic involvement. For example, the cow in **566** was scouring and recumbent, with a sunken eye exposing a congested conjunctiva. She died within a few hours as a result of toxaemia and severe dehydration.

On postmortem, the incised horn exposed necrotic cotyledons in brown, purulent fluid (567). An area of caseopurulent perimetritis is seen above the incision, with discolouration and inflammation extending over the cervix and onto the pelvic vagina (A).

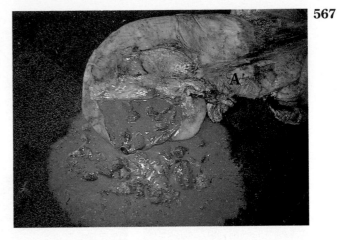

567

Vaginal prolapse

Although it may be seen after parturition, vaginal prolapse typically occurs in older cows in late pregnancy. It is associated with excess perivaginal fat, oestrogenic factors in feed leading to pelvic ligament relaxation, and with certain beef breeds, particularly Herefords. The fresh, red appearance of the prolapse in **568** indicates that it is recent, with only mild congestion from exposure. A plug of cervical mucus is visible at the lower extremity. Prolonged cases become engorged and irritant, stimulating straining. Prolapse of the vaginal wall with dystocia, as in **569**, is uncommon. The vagina is the large everted structure protruding from the vulva and ending at the cervix (A). The foetus is still within the placenta, its forefoot being palpable through the partially dilated cervix.

568

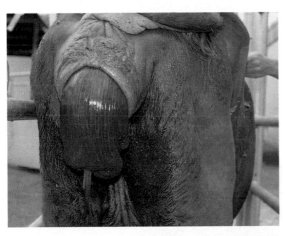

569

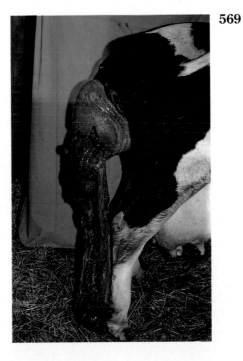

Cervical prolapse

Cervical prolapse is similar in aetiology to vaginal prolapse. Small portions of the external os of the cervix may protrude through the vulva in cows in late pregnancy or early lactation (**570**), often disappearing when they stand. A more advanced case is shown in the post-partum Shorthorn cow in **571**. The external os is oedematous and grossly distended. A short length of vaginal wall is exposed between the cervix and vulva. Complete cervicovaginal prolapse may occur. A cervical polyp (held in a gloved hand in **572**) may sometimes be confused with an early prolapse, as it appears at the vulval lips when the cow is recumbent. Vaginal polyps can also occur, but they differ in having a smooth, pink noncorrugated surface.

570   **571**   **572**

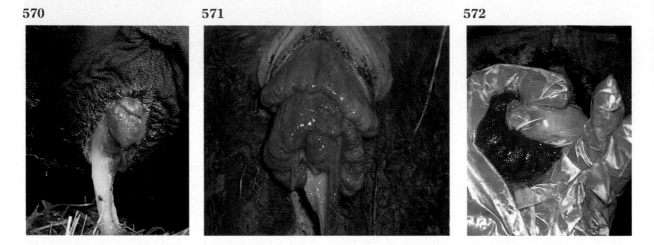

Uterine prolapse

Most cases of uterine prolapse occur within a few hours of calving. They are typically seen in older cows following dystocia or delivery of a large foetus, often associated with hypocalcaemia or a retained placenta. The young Hereford cow in **573** has a prolapse of less than two hours duration. The placenta is still attached and has a moist, fresh appearance. Most animals remain recumbent. Those which do move may traumatise the prolapse, increasing the risk of death from haemorrhage and shock. The Shorthorn cow in **574** has a complete prolapse of the uterus, vagina and cervix. This is a rare condition and, like many such cases, although the prolapse was replaced, she died within 12 hours as a result of shock and internal haemorrhage.

573

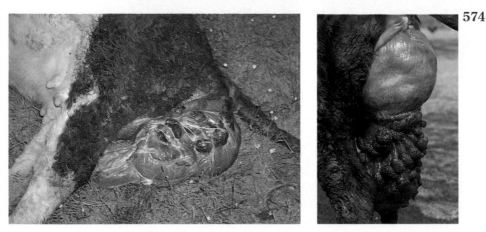

574

Abortion and premature parturition

Abortion has been defined as the premature expulsion of the products of conception, typically producing a dead calf. Premature calving occurs late in gestation, to give a live but weak calf. Both phenomena may have similar infectious and noninfectious causes. Possible infectious factors include brucellosis, IBR, BVD, leptospirosis, *Campylobacter*, bluetongue, listeriosis, *Chlamydia*, *Coxiella* and aspergillosis. Noninfectious factors include stress, lethal genes (e.g., arthrogryposis), poisons (e.g., locoweed (**716**) and mycotoxins), nutritional deficiencies (e.g., vitamin E, selenium or iodine (**67**)) and physical injuries. The appearance of an aborted foetus (the foetus in **575** was aborted at seven months of gestation) may give little indication of the cause. Specific diagnostic tests are necessary, but despite careful investigation, the cause of abortion is found in less than 25% of all cases.

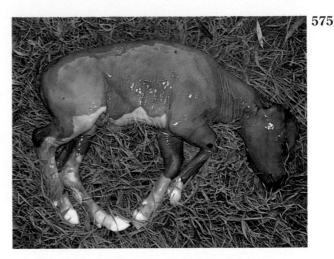

575

Premature calf

In addition to a reduced body size, the premature (seven months) Simmental crossbred calf in **576** shows hyperaemia (reddening) of the mouth and nostrils, soft hooves and a short, 'staring' coat. Most causes of abortion mentioned previously can also produce premature births. In this case, leptospirosis was the most probable. The dam had a titre of 1:1600 to *Leptospira hardjo*.

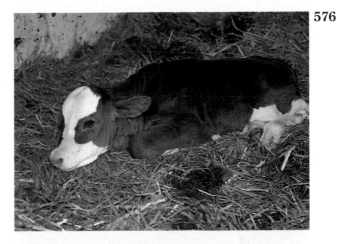

576

Mummified foetus

The foetus in **577** died at approximately four months of gestation, but was not expelled until eight months. Note the sunken eye sockets and the characteristic dry, chocolate-brown colour of the decomposing foetus and placenta. BVD is one cause of mummification. Certain bulls, especially Jerseys, may genetically produce an increased incidence of mummified foetuses.

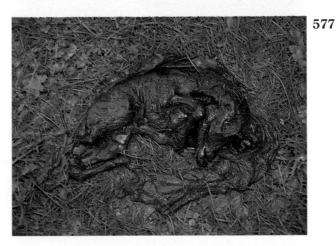

577

Brucellosis (contagious abortion)

578

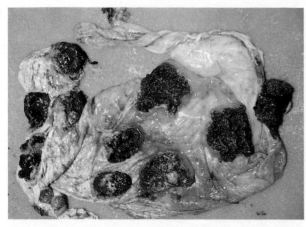

Brucellosis is a bacterial infection caused by *Brucella abortus*. Susceptible cattle ingest material from an infected foetus, placenta or uterine discharge and typically abort between seven and eight months of gestation. A marked placentitis may occur, which is seen as small, white, necrotic foci on the cotyledons and thickening of the intercotyledonary placenta (**578**). Most cows only abort once, although they may remain persistent carriers and excrete *Brucella* at subsequent normal parturitions. Retained placenta, endometritis and infertility are common complications. In the bull, the testicles (**524**) and seminal vesicles may be affected, although infection is only rarely present in the semen. Brucellosis is transmissible to humans, and is a notifiable disease in many countries.

Mycotic abortion

The mouldy silage in **579** was fed to twenty cows in late pregnancy. Haematogenous spread, leading to foetal infection, produced three abortions in ten days. *Aspergillus* was isolated from the foetuses. In some cases, small, circular, ringworm-like lesions (**580**) are seen on the foetal skin. There may also be a pronounced thickening of the placenta and necrosis of the cotyledons. *Mucor* species may also be involved.

579

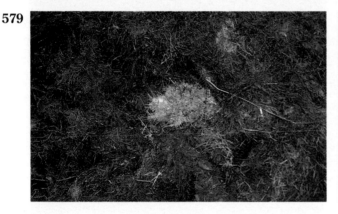

580

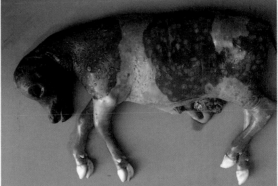

11 Udder and teat disorders

Introduction

The dairy cow is bred and fed to produce large volumes of milk. With the metabolic stress of high performance and the physical effects of being milked and handled two or three times daily, it is not surprising that the udder and teats are subject to a wide variety of disorders. The primary disease, mastitis, is of worldwide economic importance and much money is spent on its prevention, treatment and control. The first part of the chapter deals with mastitis in lactating and dry cows, and describes changes that may be seen in milk. The second part illustrates teat lesions, including a wide variety of viral infections, notably bovine herpes mammillitis, cowpox and pseudocowpox, vesicular stomatitis and fibropapillomas (warts). Other systemic diseases that also affects the teats, for example, foot-and-mouth disease, are mentioned elsewhere.

Because of their anatomical position, especially in cows with pendulous udders, teats are vulnerable to injuries, eczema and other physical influences. These problems are considered in the third part, although changes associated with photosensitisation are covered elsewhere (**72**). The final part of the chapter includes miscellaneous conditions of the udder.

Summer mastitis

Summer mastitis is an endemic form of suppurative mastitis that typically occurs sporadically in dry cows and heifers in mid–late summer. It may also arise atypically from a teat sphincter injury in a lactating cow. Mild cases become only slightly ill, whilst the more severely affected cows are dull, pyrexic and anorexic. They may abort, or produce weakly calves at term. Acute, untreated cases may die. Very few quarters recover, although cases are very occasionally mild enough to pass unrecognised until calving, when the affected quarter is nonfunctional ('blind') (see also **590**) and the teat is palpably thickened.

The Charolais heifer in **581** is an early case, showing distension of the left hind quarter, which was typically hard and sore, with a prominent, turgid teat. Several bacteria are involved, including *Actinomyces (Corynebacterium) pyogenes*, *Peptococcus indolicus*, *Streptococcus dysgalactiae* and a micrococcus which contributes to the typical odour. Infection is thought to be transmitted by the head fly *Hydrotoea irritans*. In more advanced cases, the infection may burst through the udder, as shown in the right hind quarter in **582**. A thickening of the central teat canal was palpable, the quarter was very hard, and yellow pus with a pungent odour was discharging from the teat and udder. Control of summer mastitis includes dry cow therapy with long-acting intramammary antibiotics, fly repellents, and keeping cattle away from known fly areas.

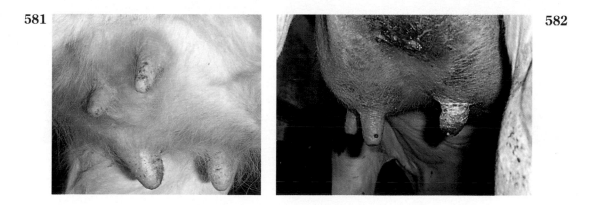

581

582

Acute mastitis

Peracute and acute mastitis are most commonly seen in the first few weeks after calving, although cases can occur throughout lactation. In most cases, peracute mastitis results from coliform or staphylococcal infections. Similarly, in acute mastitis, environmental organisms such as coliforms (e.g., *Escherichia coli*) or *Streptococcus uberis* are frequently involved. Infection enters the teat and the udder between milkings. Acute disease may occasionally be caused by 'contagious' mastitis organisms such as staphylococci, which are carried on the skin or in the udder of affected cows and transmitted to other cows during milking.

The most prominent sign of acute mastitis is an enlarged, hard, hot and painful quarter. This may be apparent before any changes are visible in the milk. In some cases, a brown serous discharge may be seen on the surface of the affected quarter and teat, as in the lactating Friesian cow in **583**. In a section of an affected udder (**584**), deep red inflammation of the teat cistern and teat canal mucosa is seen. There is prominent subcutaneous oedema and the skin at the tip of the teat is congested. Changes of this nature can lead to gangrene. The yellow foci (A) in the udder parenchyma are pockets of pus. In **585** the teat skin, which was still warm and soft, and the affected quarter, are encircled by a ring of black gangrene, with red erythema at the periphery. The cow was severely ill with an eventually fatal toxaemia.

Such cases should not be confused with udder bruising (**586**). In this cow the forequarter is obviously enlarged, the front teat deviates medially, and a blue discolouration is seen on the lower half of both quarters. The cow was, however, bright and alert, there were no visible changes in the milk, and the skin remained warm.

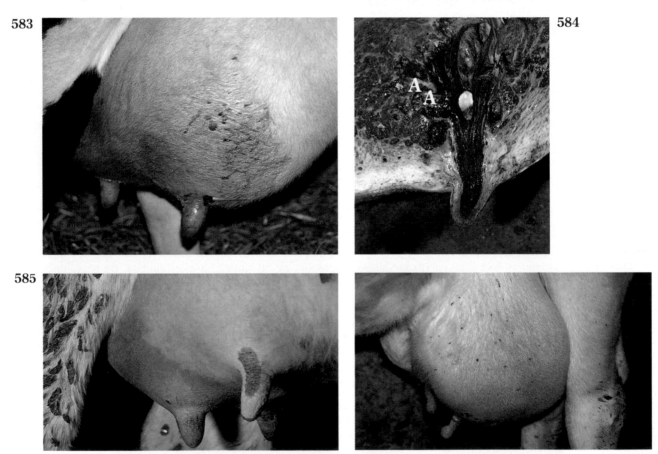

583

584

585

58

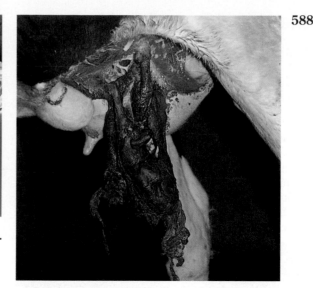

Advanced gangrene (**587**) leads to cold, damp teat skin. Although mastitis was limited to the right hind quarter (A), the entire udder was blue, oedematous, and cold to the touch. Adjacent to the affected teat is a skin slough and red exudate. The secretion from the udder was a deep port-wine colour and was mixed with gas. The cow had been normal when milked 12 hours previously, indicating the sudden onset of disease. In cases of nonfatal, gangrenous mastitis the overlying skin (**588**), or even the entire affected quarter, sloughs in a process which may take 1–2 months.

Chronic mastitis and blind quarter

Streptococcus agalactiae, Strep. dysgalactiae, staphylococci, *Corynebacterium bovis* and other bacteria can produce a chronic mastitis, manifested as 'clots' in the milk (**593**), with or without palpable udder changes.

Carrier cows act as a reservoir of infection and bacteria are transmitted to other quarters or other cows during milking. Hygiene, teat disinfection, correct milking machine function, dry cow antibiotic therapy and culling are important control measures. The Friesian cow in **589** shows large, hard nodules protruding from the udder, with two from the right quarter and one from the left. These are chronic, intramammary, staphylococcal abscesses. Staphylococci were cultured from the milk, which had a high cell count and gave a strongly positive reaction to the California mastitis test. Such advanced cases, which are usually unresponsive to treatment, are dangerous carriers and should be culled. The Friesian cow in **590** had a blind quarter, having had mastitis in the previous lactation. The front left teat is slightly smaller than the others, and the associated quarter has totally atrophied. Blind quarters in heifers with nonpatent teats can be either congenital (total absence of the teat canal or persistence of membrane between the cistern and canal at the teat base), or acquired, e.g., undetected summer mastitis, when a thickened central core is palpable in the teat canal, or trauma from being suckled as a calf (**39**).

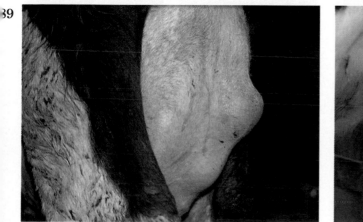

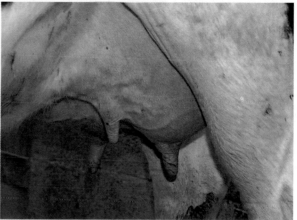

Mastitic changes in milk

Milk is thicker and more viscous during the dry period and immediately postpartum (i.e., colostrum). Its character also changes in mastitis. Although specific types of mastitic infection frequently lead to similar changes in milk, the appearance of the milk is *not* pathognomonic, and bacteriological examination is required to confirm the causative organism and to determine the antibiotic sensitivity.

Blood in milk

True blood clots are the characteristic feature of blood in milk. They may be present in slightly pink-tinged milk (**591**) or, in more severe cases, in a secretion that is almost totally red (**592**). Seen only in newly-calved cows, or after trauma, the condition usually resolves spontaneously. No treatment has been found to be consistently useful. Herd outbreaks of unknown aetiology may occur.

591

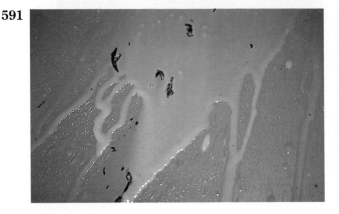

59

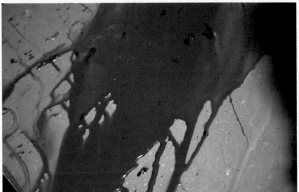

Mastitic milk

Watery, translucent milk with occasional clots (**593**) is typical of a mild mastitis such as that caused by *Streptococcus agalactiae* or *Strep. dysgalactiae*. Normal milk may be totally absent in severe staphylococcal (**594**) or *Actinomyces (Corynebacterium) pyogenes* infections, when the secretion consists of thick clots suspended in a clear, serous fluid. Summer mastitis (*Actinomyces*) invariably produces a thick secretion with a characteristic pungent odour.

A brownish, serum-coloured secretion is typical of *Escherichia coli* infection (**595**), while acute gangrenous mastitis (e.g., acute staphylococcal) may produce a red or brown homogenous secretion (**596**), often mixed with gas.

593 **594** **595** **596**

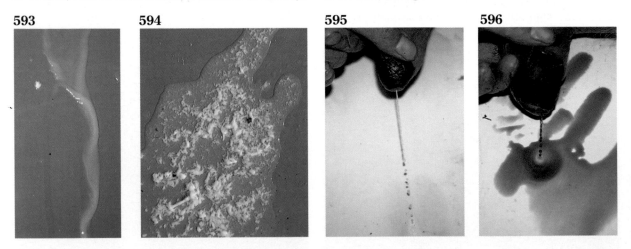

Infectious teat conditions

Teats are affected by two pox viruses, pseudocowpox (paravaccinia), a mild infection that occurs throughout the world, and cowpox (vaccinia), which is now extremely rare. Both are transmissible to man. The parapoxvirus of pseudocowpox is related to bovine papular stomatitis (**143 & 144**). Bovine herpes mammillitis is a much more severe infection and may be confused clinically with the teat changes associated with necrotic dermatitis (udder seborrhoea). Other viral infections producing teat lesions include vesic-ular stomatitis (**604**), fibropapillomas (**605–607**), bluetongue (**643**), foot and mouth disease (**629**) and rinderpest (**634**). Teats are also subject to physical injury, chapping and eczema often exacerbated by cold, wet conditions, twice daily milking and poor milking machine function. Examples include hyperkeratosis and 'black spot' of the teat sphincter (**608**), summer (licking) sores (**614**), trauma, and photosensitisation (**72**).

Bovine herpes mammillitis

Bovine herpes mammillitis (BHM) is a viral infection that initially produces fluid-filled vesicles, seen in the centre and towards the tip of the teat in **597**. The overlying epithelium is stretched and white. Rupture of the initial vesicles exposes raw, ulcerated areas (seen between the two vesicles in **597**), which later become covered by thick, brown scabs (**598**). Note the involvement of three teats and the extension of the le-sions onto the udder skin. The condition is so painful that it is often impossible to milk affected cows (compare pseudocowpox, **599–602**). BHM tends to occur in outbreaks and secondary mastitis is a major problem. Lifelong immunity follows recovery. *Differential diagnosis*: necrotic dermatitis (**622–625**) and bluetongue (**643**).

597

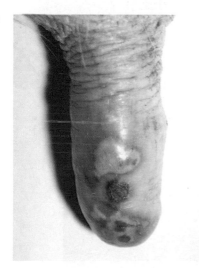

598

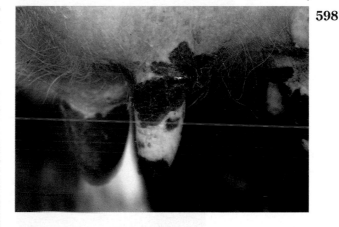

Pseudocowpox (paravaccinia)

Pseudocowpox is caused by a parapox virus and is a common infection in many parts of the world, spreading slowly within a herd. Both the teats (primarily) and the udder may be affected and 'milker's nodules' may occur on the fingers of man. An individual cow may remain clinically affected for several months and, as immunity is short-lived, repeated attacks can occur every 2–3 years. The disease starts as a small, painless papule affecting the superficial layers of the skin (**599**). After 7–10 days the lesion enlarges from the periphery to produce characteristic circular or horseshoe-shaped areas, delineated by small, red scabs (**600**). The affected area feels rough, but is not painful, and milking is not usually impeded. Scabs slowly resolve in the healing phase (**601**). In rare cases, the lesion develops a very rough, slightly moist, papilliform appearance, with several elevated and confluent masses (**602**). *Differential diagnosis*: bluetongue (**641**), cowpox (**603**), and vesicular stomatitis (**604**).

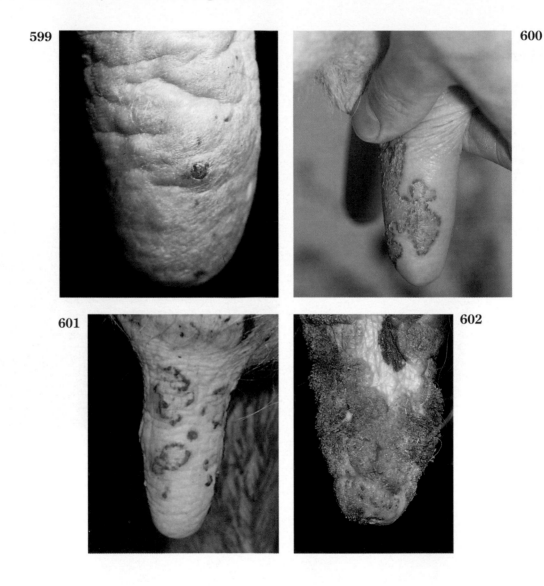

599 600 601 602

Cowpox (vaccinia)

Caused by a pox virus closely related to smallpox in man, cowpox produces vesicles on the skin of the teats and the udder. **603** illustrates three teat skin vesicles which have ruptured, exposing the underlying granulation tissue. Cowpox is now extremely rare and the infection is limited to Western Europe.

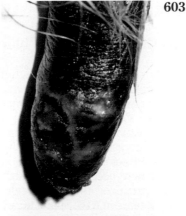

603

Vesicular stomatitis

Vesicular stomatitis is caused by a rhabdovirus that is found only in North and South America and is transmitted by mosquitoes and biting flies. It primarily produces mouth lesions (**141**), but lesions can also occur on the teats and coronet. Multiple, irregular-shaped, white vesicles, some of which have ruptured, cover much of the teat skin in **604**. Recovered animals are immune for 12–18 months.

604

Fibropapillomas (warts)

Caused by different strains of papovaviruses, warts are common among groups of pregnant and first lactation heifers, typically over the lower part of the teat. Some have a 'feathery', keratinised and papilliform appearance (**605**) and can be easily pulled off. Others are more nodular (**606**) and tightly adherent to the skin. Mixed infections may occur (**607**). Fibropapillomas close to the teat orifice and sphincter interfere with milking and predispose animals to teat stenosis and mastitis. Flies are considered to be important vectors for transmission. Autogenous vaccines are generally more effective than commercial. Warts also occur on the skin (**100**), eye (**450**) and penis (**510**).

605 606 607

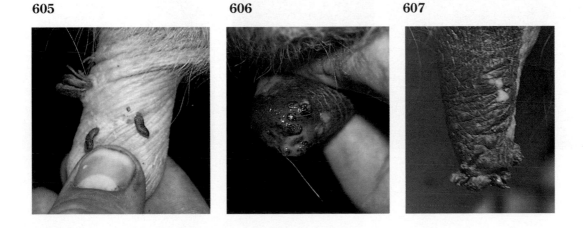

Noninfectious teat conditions

Teat orifice lesions (hyperkeratosis, 'black spot', chaps and fissures)

Hyperkeratosis is initially seen as a raised, pale, bulbous swelling of the circular sphincter area, with small, protruding fragments of dry, keratinised material (**608**). Advanced cases, which predispose to mastitis, show severe keratinisation (**609**), which may precede black spot. Although associated with faulty milking machine function, other factors are also involved and the condition may occur spontaneously. Milking machine trauma produced the dry, circular, haemorrhagic areas on the teats in **610**. Sphincter eversion is marked.

Black spot or black pox describes a proliferative necrotic dermatitis of the teat end around the sphincter, seen extending to the left in **611**. Black necrotic tissue is clearly visible. The lesion is caused by a range of environmental traumas (e.g., overmilking, excessive vacuum fluctuation, wet teats exposed to a chilling wind), leading to damage of the teat orifice, which may then become secondarily infected with *Fusobacterium necrophorum*. The skin fissure adjacent to the black spot lesion in **611** is a teat chap, which often results from repeated exposure to wet, cold winds or, sometimes, to irritant chemicals. It is not unusual for the whole teat to be affected (**612**). Severe skin fissures or teat chaps (**613**) can sometimes virtually obliterate the teat orifice. Topical emollients are important in prevention.

608 **609** **610**

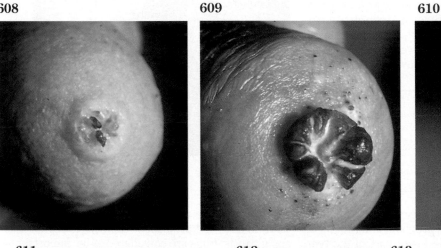

611 **612** **613**

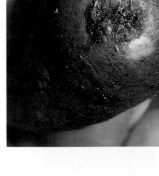
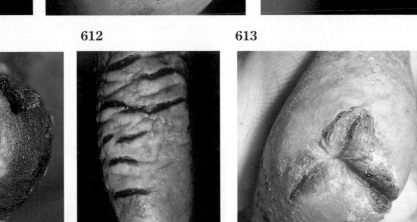

Summer sores and teat eczema

Summer sores are eczematous lesions that result from excessive licking, and may be secondary to irritation caused by flies. First seen as irregular-shaped areas of moist, wet eczema at the teat base, they may spread to involve almost the entire teat (**614**), when they can be very painful. **614** shows islets of residual epithelium in the granulation tissue, especially towards the tip of the teat, and there is a serous exudate. At this stage, differential diagnosis from bovine herpes mammillitis (**598**) and necrotic dermatitis (**622**) is difficult. Simple sunburn producing a thickening of teat skin may also occur (**71**).

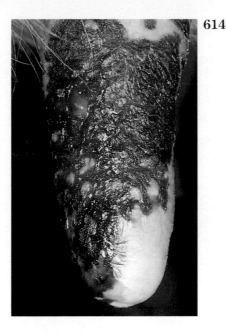

614

Teat trauma

Because of their position, teats are very prone to injury, especially in cows with turgid or pendulous udders. Barbed wire often produces multiple lacerations and may leave a horizontal flap of skin (**615**). This flap tends to be pulled downwards when the teat cups are removed at milking, thus retarding healing. Amputation of the skin flap promotes healing. Superficial epidermal abrasions (**616**) cause few problems, although this teat had been injured in a previous lactation, leaving a fistula (A) of the cistern at its base. Trauma can cause complete loss of a large area of skin, but this often heals surprisingly well. Injuries such as a contaminated flap involving the teat sphincter, or localised ulceration (**617**), carry a high risk of both mastitis and stenosis of the orifice.

615

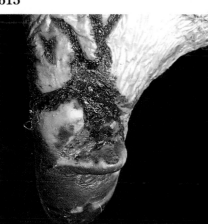

616

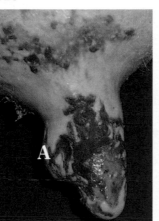

A

617

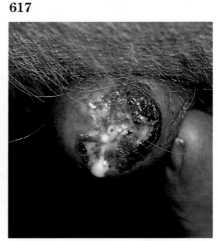

Teat cistern granuloma ('pea')

Free-floating, irregular, rubbery masses of fibrocollagenous material ('peas') may develop in the teat cistern and pass down to the sphincter, thus obstructing the milk flow. As in **618**, some can be manually expressed from a surgically dilated teat orifice. Others

are attached to the teat mucosa and cannot be so easily removed. A variety of shapes, sizes and colours is found (**619**). All have a rubbery texture and are 5–10 mm long.

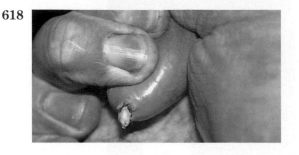

618

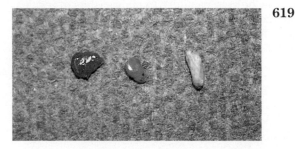

619

Supernumerary teats

Supernumerary teats are a congenital condition. They may be found between the front and rear teats, and/or attached to the udder behind the rear teats (**620**), or to the base or side of one of the main teats, where they can interfere with milking. Typically, they are shorter than normal teats, and have thinner walls. They may connect to the sinus of an existing teat, or, more commonly, have a separate supernumerary gland. As such teats are both unsightly and may develop mastitis, they are normally removed early in life, when extreme care is necessary to identify the correct teat.

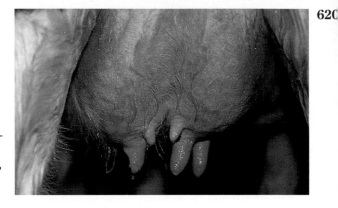

620

Conditions of the udder skin and subcutis

Udder impetigo (udder acne)

Small, red papules are seen on the udder of the Friesian in **621**. They sometimes coalesce to produce an exudative dermatitis that can spread onto the teats and may develop a foul odour. A coagulase-positive staphylococcus was isolated in this case. Topical therapy is effective. *Differential diagnosis* (of advanced teat cases): bovine herpes mammillitis (**597**) and necrotic dermatitis (**622**).

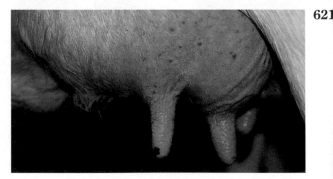

621

Necrotic dermatitis (udder seborrhoea)

This dermatitis occurs in the first 1–2 weeks after calving, especially in heifers, and is associated with excessive prepartum udder oedema, leading to skin ischaemia and necrosis. Mild cases (**622**) develop a moist and often foul-smelling superficial dermatitis laterally in the contact area between the udder and thigh. In more advanced cases (**623**) the ischaemic udder skin turns reddish-purple and produces a dirty, serous exudate, similar to some cases of acute or peracute mastitis (**583**). A dry, scaly dermatitis (**624**) may lead to extensive thickening of the teats, and some animals become impossible to milk. Note the residual cutaneous oedema cranial to the udder in this heifer.

In mature cows the usual site of the dermatitis is the area of skin between the two forequarters and the ventral body wall. The lesion, which may persist for several weeks, is a deep, moist and exudative dermatitis with a pungent odour (**625**). Necrotic debris is seen in the centre. *Differential diagnosis*: severe udder impetigo (staphylococcal dermatitis) (**621**), bluetongue (**643**), bovine herpes mammillitis (**597**).

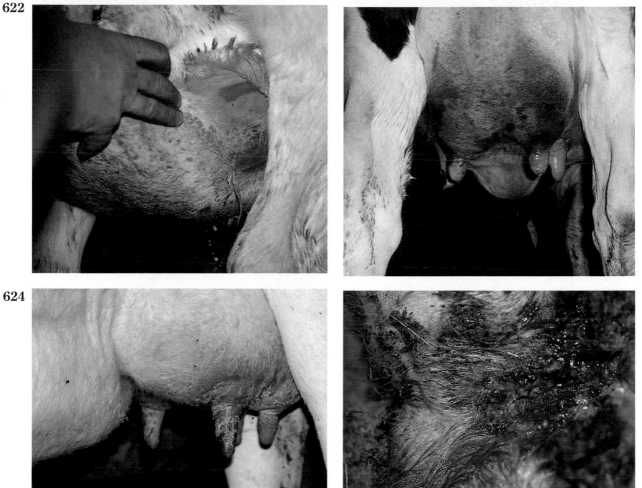

622

623

624

625

Ventral abdominal oedema

A physiological periparturient condition, extensive subcutaneous oedema is seen cranial to the udder of the Holstein heifer in **626**, two days after calving. In advanced cases it may extend to the sternum.

Typically, oedema is demonstrated as 'pitting' when pressure is applied. Digital pressure on the rear of an oedematous udder (**627**) creates a depression (seen to the left of the finger (A)) which persists for 30–60 seconds after the finger has been withdrawn. Overfeeding, an overfat prepartum condition, heredity and lack of exercise are among the factors contributing to excess oedema.

626

627

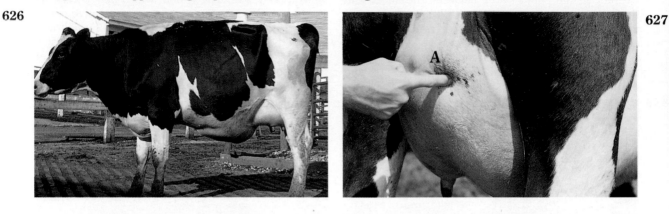

Dropped udder (rupture of median suspensory apparatus)

The six-year-old Guernsey cow in **628** had calved four weeks previously, and had suddenly developed a grossly pendulous udder as a result of sudden rupture of the median suspensory apparatus (ligaments) of the udder. Note that the ventral udder surface is considerably below the level of the hock. The outward direction of the teats is a mechanical result of the loss of ligamentous support of the udder, which had no evidence of mastitis. Postmortem examination revealed a massive haematoma surrounding the ligamentous rupture between the ventral body wall and the gland parenchyma. Breeding and prepartum overfeeding that leads to excessive udder engorgement are predisposing factors. *Differential diagnosis*: acute mastitis, ventral abdominal rupture (prepubic tendon (**121**), or rectus abdominis muscle) and severe udder oedema (**627**).

628

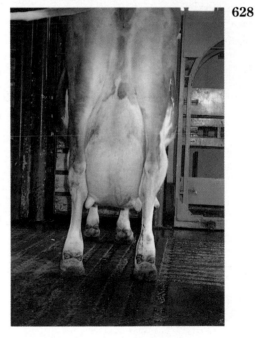

12 Infectious diseases

Introduction

Infectious diseases are a major limiting factor in cattle production in many parts of the world. In tropical Africa, with its 161 million cattle, the major diseases, i.e., rinderpest, foot-and-mouth disease, contagious bovine pleuropneumonia, theileriosis and trypanosomiasis, are all infectious. Such limitations on livestock production lead to shortages of meat, milk, draught animals and manure, and to the necessity to import from developed countries such as North America and Australia, and the European Community. These imports in turn discourage domestic livestock production, while the presence of infectious diseases bars the export of cattle and cattle products to the developed countries.

Viral diseases

Several major bovine diseases, endemic in many parts of the world, have a viral aetiology. They are characterised by their highly contagious nature and the variety of their cloven-footed hosts. Early recognition of suspicious signs and confirmation of the disease in the laboratory, together with prompt and effective control measures, are essential for their eradication.

Foot-and-mouth disease (FMD)

Cattle infected with foot-and-mouth disease are dull, off feed, and drool saliva. Some are lame. On opening the mouth (**629**), large areas of epithelial loss, that are the result of recently ruptured FMD vesicles, are seen on the tongue and hard palate, as in this animal from Zimbabwe.

629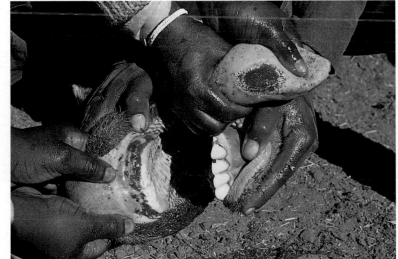

In a steer infected experimentally two days previously, ulcers are seen along the lower gums and inside the lower lip, together with ruptured tongue vesicles (**630**). Two days later the lesions on the tongue, lower lip and gums have become secondarily infected (**631**). On the fifth day, vesicles on the coronary band and dorsal part of the interdigital space have ruptured (**632**), and on the seventh (**633**) the interdigital space shows widespread ulceration along its entire length. Lameness may be the first sign of FMD. These interdigital lesions easily become secondarily infected. *Differential diagnosis:* includes vesicular stomatitis (**141**), BVD/MD (**132**), bovine papular stomatitis (**143** & **144**) and rinderpest (**636**).

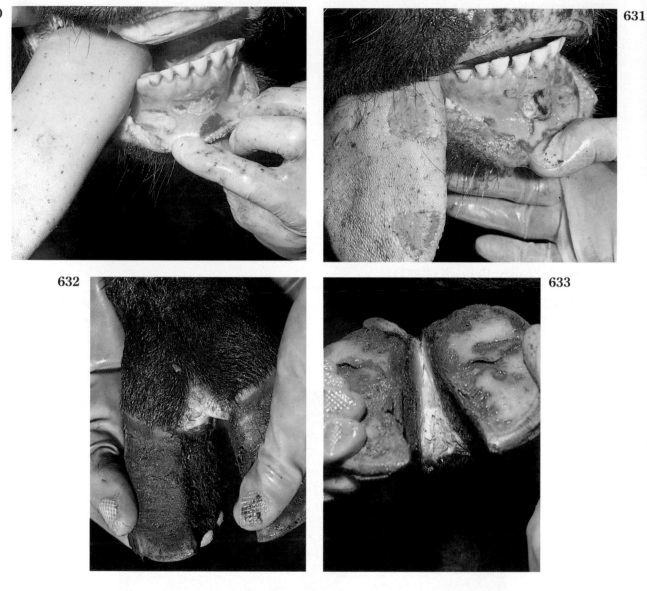

630

631

632

633

Rinderpest ('cattle plague')

Rinderpest is a very severe, contagious disease with a mortality of up to 100%, especially when outbreaks occur in previously free areas (**634**). It is endemic in parts of Africa, the Middle East and the Indian subcontinent. Multinational campaigns to eradicate rinderpest from West and Central Africa have failed in many cases, despite the initial successful use of an effective vaccine. Various factors have been to blame, including wars, a shortage of trained personnel, lack of refrigeration for storage of vaccines, and other organisational problems. Early recognition and notification of outbreaks of rinderpest are vital to any eradication campaign. The causal agent, a paramyxovirus, causes a severe oculonasal discharge, which may become purulent (eye **635**, nares **636**) with necrosis and diph-

theresis. An early oral sign, seen within 2–3 days of infection, is the formation of small, pinpoint areas of necrosis on the ventral (never the dorsal) surface of the tongue (**637**) which develop into plaques within 1–2 days. These are also seen on the gums and dental pad in **638**. Necrotic and erosive lesions extend along

634

635

636

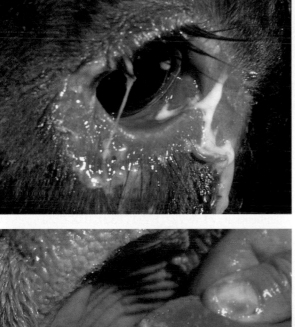

637

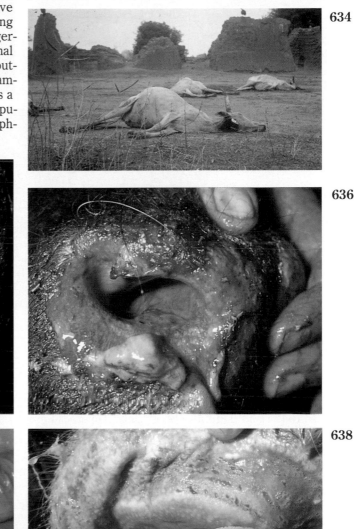

638

the entire length of the alimentary tract, from the hard palate to the pharynx and oesophagus (**639**), and the typical zebra-striped rectum in **640**, leading to severe diarrhoea and death from dehydration. Lesions are indistinguishable clinically from BVD (**132**), and other differential diagnoses include IBR (**222**) and malignant catarrhal fever (**644**). The illustrations are from Saudi Arabia, Yemen and Nigeria.

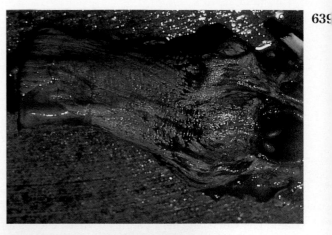

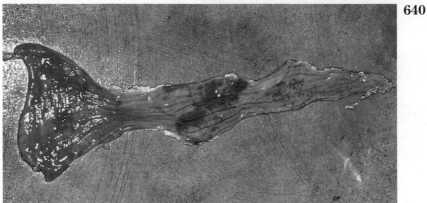

640

Bluetongue

Bluetongue causes initial hyperaemia of the muzzle and lips (**641**), followed by inflammatory and erosive lesions. Necrotic areas may be seen in the gums and the dental pad (**642**), and there may be irregular, superficial erosions on the teats (**643**). The disease is caused by an orbivirus and is transmitted by biting insects (*Culicoides*). While endemic on the African continent, blue-

tongue is sporadic in many other parts of the world. In North America it is a mild clinical condition and differential diagnosis is difficult. It has been mistaken for photosensitisation (**71 & 72**), BVD (**132**), IBR (**223**), vesicular stomatitis (**141**) and FMD (**629**). Mycotic stomatitis is also caused by the bluetongue virus.

641 **642** **643**

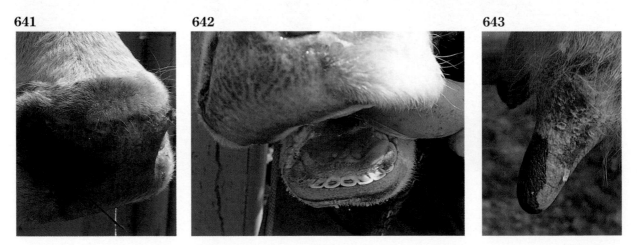

Malignant catarrhal fever (MCF, bovine malignant catarrh, malignant head catarrh)

Malignant catarrhal fever causes a severe pyrexia with catarrhal and mucopurulent inflammation of the upper respiratory and alimentary epithelia, keratoconjunctivitis following a characteristic initial peripheral keratitis, and lymphadenopathy. MCF outbreaks occur predominantly in Africa. Elsewhere (North America and Europe), single individuals tend to show signs. The 'head and eye' syndrome of the Devon cow in **644** includes a purulent oculonasal discharge, mild keratitis, and hyperaemia of the nostrils. After a few days, dried material becomes caked on the nostrils (**645**). The peripheral keratitis is demonstrated in **646**. Iridocyclitis may lead to photophobia. Areas of haemorrhagic necrosis and ulceration (**647**) are particularly prominent in the oral and nasal cavities (A). MCF is almost invariably fatal and no vaccine regime is currently available. Clinical cases should be isolated. *Differential diagnosis*: rinderpest (**634**), bluetongue (**641**), East Coast fever (**665**), IBR (**222**), BVD/MD (**130**) and bovine iritis (**443**).

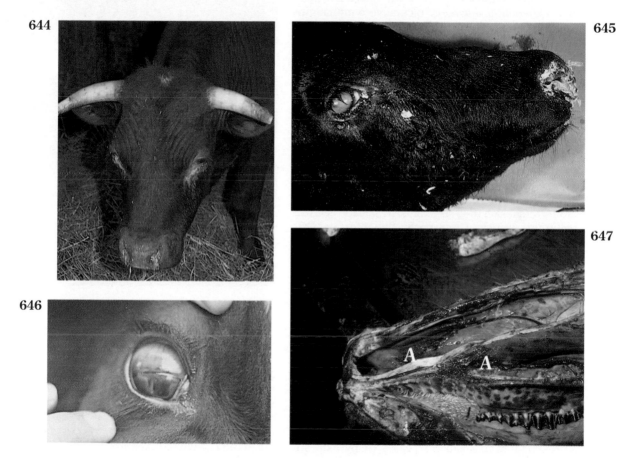

644

645

646

647

Lumpy-skin disease

An infectious disease that is limited to Africa, lumpy-skin disease produces nodules on the skin and elsewhere, which may become secondarily infected. The nodules (648) are discrete, firm, raised and painful masses involving the skin, as well as the gastrointestinal, respiratory and genital tracts (orchitis), and the conjunctiva. The nodules contain firm, grey-yellow material. The regional lymph nodes are enlarged (prescapular in 648). There are two distinct diseases, one of which is caused by the 'Neethling' poxvirus, while the milder form is due to infection with the 'Allerton' herpesvirus. *Differential diagnosis:* ulcerative lymphangitis (pseudotuberculosis) (102), pseudo-lumpy-skin disease and streptothricosis (dermatophilosis) (97).

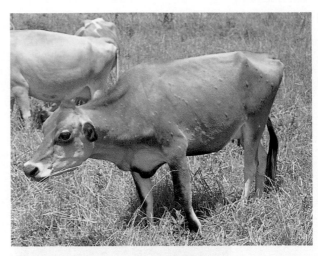

Rift Valley fever

Rift Valley fever (RVF) is confined to Africa, with epizootics occurring in southern and central Africa, and more recently in Egypt. It is an acute febrile disease that is communicable to humans. The cause is a phlebovirus (Bunyaviridae). Affected calves usually die after a short illness, but abortion is the main clinical sign in adult cattle, which have a lower mortality rate. The characteristic postmortem lesion (649) is extensive hepatic necrosis, seen in this section of an experimental infection. Diagnosis rests on laboratory serological testing. In the absence of a vaccine, control depends on strict prohibition of the importation of susceptible cattle from endemic parts of the African continent. *Differential diagnosis*: bluetongue (641) and rinderpest (634).

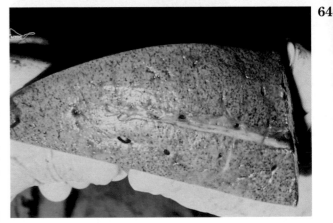

Ephemeral fever ('three-day sickness')

Severe cases of ephemeral fever are initially seen in sternal recumbency and later in lateral recumbency (650) with signs of flaccid paralysis. Other features include rumen atony, loss of the swallow reflex and tongue tonus (651), and partial paralysis of the lower jaw, resembling botulism. Mild cases are pyrexic, stiff and only slightly ill. The disease occurs in Africa, Asia and Australia, and is caused by an insect-borne (e.g., sandfly) rhabdovirus. Other signs include fever, muscle stiffness, lameness, atypical interstitial pneumonia, and lymphadenopathy. *Differential diagnosis*: botulism (687), severe toxaemia, physical injury.

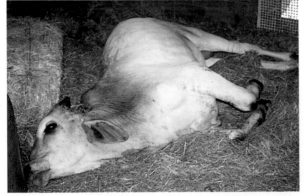

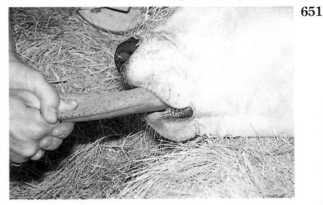

Tick-borne diseases (protozoal and rickettsial infections)

In tropical Africa, ticks are very important owing to their impact on the cattle industry. Tick infestations depress productivity as a direct result of their feeding activity. This is primarily through reduced liveweight gain, and other consequences including anaemia, skin wounds that are susceptible to secondary bacterial infection or screw-worm infestation (**110**), and toxic reactions to tick saliva (e.g., sweating sickness, **670** & **671**). Indirectly however, they have a far more significant role as vectors of diseases such as East Coast fever (ECF) and theileriosis throughout East and Southern Africa, where they cause the death of half a million cattle each year in the endemic areas.

Other tick-borne diseases that limit cattle production in Africa and elsewhere include babesiosis, anaplasmosis, heartwater (cowdriosis) and streptothricosis. Ticks parasitic on cattle can be divided into two families, the Ixodidae or 'hard' ticks and the Argasidae or 'soft' ticks, depending on the presence or absence of a hard, dorsal scutum. These families also have many other differences.

Tick infestations

652

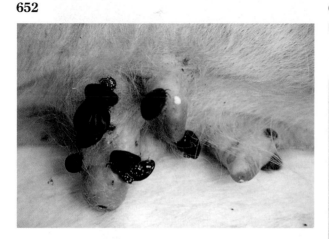

653   **654**

Taken in Antigua, West Indies, **652** shows *Amblyomma variegatum* ticks feeding on teats. These species are mainly found in the tropics and subtropics, causing disease both directly and by parasite transmission. Mixed tick infections do occur. Their large mouthparts can cause serious wounds that are liable to secondary infection. The scrotum is also a common region for tick feeding. In **653** *Amblyomma* species (bont ticks) are seen in varying stages of engorgement, feeding around the perineum and anus of a four-month-old Friesian heifer from Zimbabwe. White larvae along the edge of the tail indicate early myiasis lesions. These changes are more pronounced in **654**, where tick damage has resulted in an enlarged vulva, with raw, bleeding areas. Early myiasis is again visible. Myiasis lesions are also shown in **110** and **111**.

Babesiosis ('redwater fever')

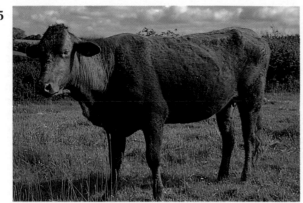

655

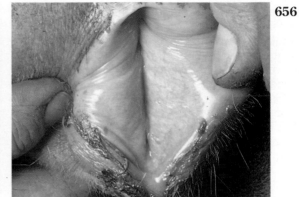

656

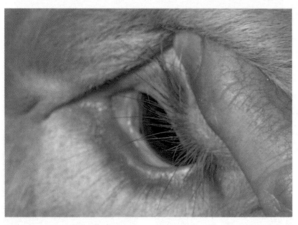

657

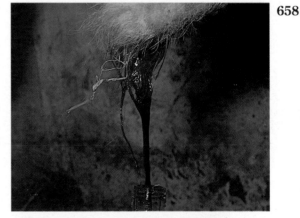

658

The term 'redwater' originates from the haemoglobinuria that is seen following a haemolytic anaemia produced by protozoa of *Babesia* species, *B. bovis* and *B. divergens* being the most important. They may occur singly or together, and in combination with *Anaplasma* to produce fatal 'tick fever'. The South Devon cow in **655** has lost condition. She has a dejected appearance, with drooping ears, half-closed eyes and the front legs abducted to maintain balance. Her flank is hollow, indicating lack of rumen fill. There is extreme pallor of the vulval membranes (**656**) and the conjunctiva is both anaemic and jaundiced (**657**). Dark, port wine-coloured urine, as seen in the South Devon steer in **658**, often produces a characteristic golden yellow froth as it hits the ground (**659**). Affected cattle are

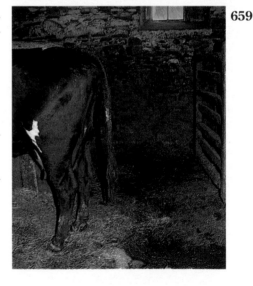

659

febrile and develop anal sphincter spasm, producing 'coiling' of faeces which are voided under pressure (**660**). *Ixodes ricinus* is the vector for *Babesia bigemina*. Disease caused by babesiosis is distributed worldwide wherever there are ticks. *Differential diagnosis* (of redwater): includes anaplasmosis (**661**), bracken poisoning (**700**), kale poisoning (**707**), bacillary haemoglobinuria and nitrate poisoning (**724**).

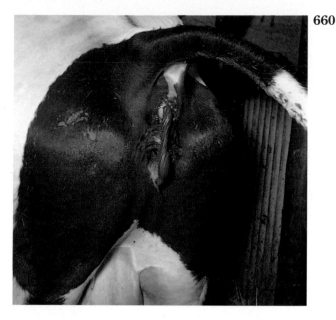

660

Anaplasmosis ('gall sickness')

Caused by the rickettsia, *Anaplasma marginale*, gall sickness is endemic in tropical and subtropical regions of Africa, Australia and the Americas. Transmission is by ticks (*Boophilus* and *Dermacentor species*), biting flies, or iatrogenically, for example, during mass vaccination. Adult cattle are more severely affected. After initial pyrexia and anorexia, anaemia develops, as shown on the vaginal mucosa in **661**, and later jaundice (**662**). Mortality may reach 50%.

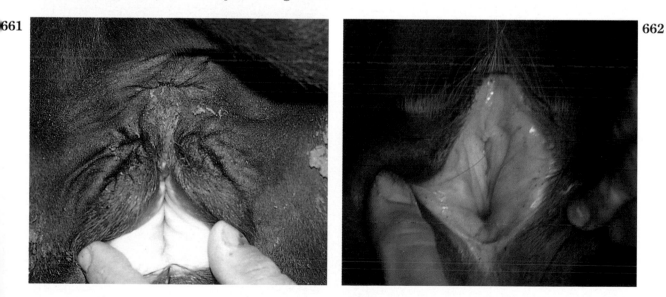

661

662

On postmortem examination (**663**), the carcase is pale, anaemic and slightly jaundiced. Unclotted blood can be seen on the hide adjacent to the spine. The liver is enlarged and mottled (**664**) and the distended gall-bladder contains thick bile, and there is splenic enlargement. Recovered animals may remain carriers for life. These illustrations are from Zimbabwe and from Queensland, Australia.

663

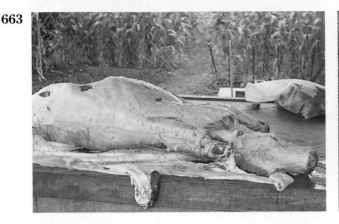

664

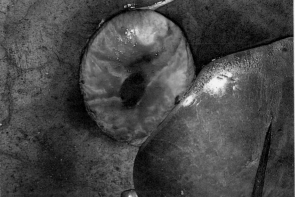

Theileriosis ('East Coast fever', ECF)

Theileria species are tick-borne protozoal parasites that multiply in lymphocytes and then enter erythrocytes. Theileriosis is common in tick-infested areas throughout the world. *T. parva* (East Coast fever, ECF), transmitted by *Rhipicephalus appendiculatus*, is a serious problem in Central and East Africa. *T. annulata*, transmitted by *Hyalomma* species, occurs in North Africa, the Middle East, India and Asia. In **665**, the Jersey heifer from Zimbabwe is in poor condition and shows gross enlargement of the parotid and prescapular lymph nodes, a rough coat (particularly dorsally), and matted hair over the face due to epiphora. Affected animals are pyrexic and anaemic. On postmortem examination, splenic enlargement severe pulmonary emphysema and oedema, and

665

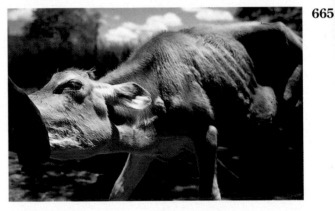

generalised lymphoid hyperplasia are the most striking changes.

Cowdriosis ('heartwater')

Caused by the rickettsial organism, *Cowdria ruminatum*, heartwater is transmitted from reservoir hosts (e.g., wildebeest) to susceptible cattle by *Amblyomma* (bont) ticks, producing severe damage to the vascular endothelium. The disease is common in many parts of Africa and the Caribbean; the cattle illustrated are from Mali. Peracute disease produces rapid death. Acute cases are initially dull, pyrexic and anorexic, with a 'tucked up' abdomen, as seen in the Zebu steer in **666**. Nervous signs, convulsions, maniacal behaviour and death in extensor spasm may follow rapidly, with a frothy discharge from the nostrils (**667**). Increased vascular permeability produces a generalised circulatory failure, seen as lung congestion, hydrothorax and hydropericardium (**668,** where the forceps raise the margin of the incised pericardium). In **669** the cut surface of an affected lung shows massive interlobular oedema (A) and congestion (B).

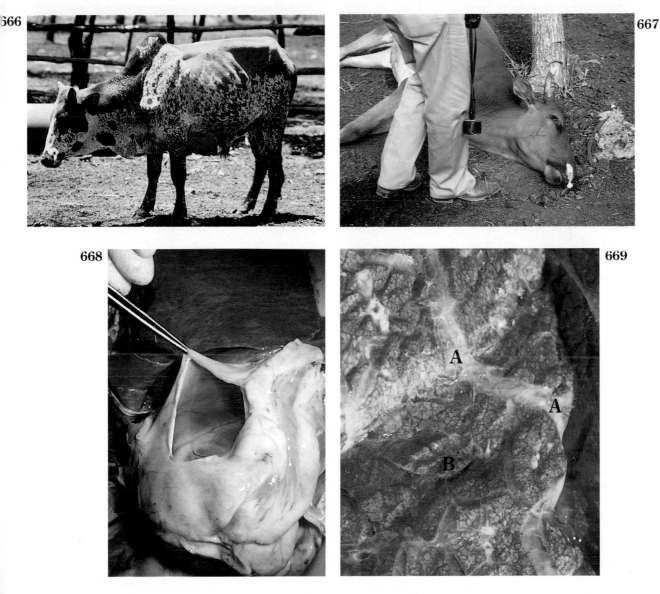

Sweating sickness

Sweating sickness is seen in Central and Southern Africa and India. The aetiology involves a toxin, produced by the female *Hyalomma truncatum* tick when she weighs 20–50 mg, resulting in toxicosis. As in the Friesian calf from Zimbabwe (**670**), the tick must feed for 5–7 days before sufficient toxin has passed into the host to produce clinical signs. The moist dermatitis (sweat) typically affects the inguinum, the perineum and the axilla, producing a sour smell. Note the early myiasis ventral to the vulva. Young calves are usually affected and immunity lasts for 4–5 years. Hair loss, which may be total, occurs secondary to the initial moist dermatitis. Hair may be pulled off when the animal is handled, for example over the ears (**671**). Lacrimation and salivation may occur because all mucous membranes are affected.

670 671

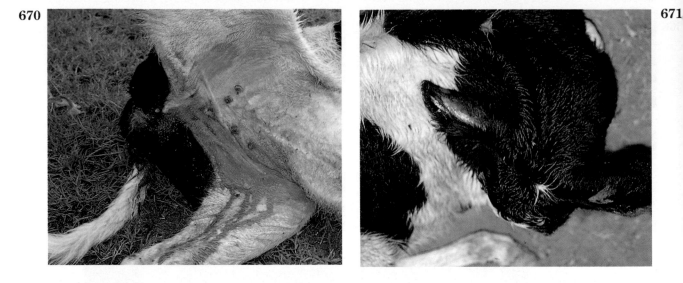

Sporadic bovine encephalomyelitis (SBE,' buss disease')

672

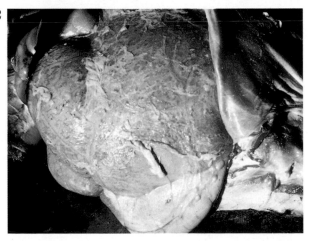

Sporadic bovine encephalomyelitis is an uncommon systemic infection, caused by *Chlamydia psittaci*. A paramyxoviral SBE, recently described, is a separate entity. Also known as transmissible necrosis, it has a worldwide distribution and causes a generalised inflammation of blood vessels, serous membranes and synoviae. The calf in **672** shows a chronic fibrinous exudative peritonitis. Pleurisy and pericarditis were also present.

Ondiri disease (bovine petechial fever, ehrlichiosis)

One characteristic feature of Ondiri disease is petechiation of mucosal surfaces, shown as haemorrhages beneath the tongue (**673**), on the epicardium (**674**) and in an affected lymph node (**675**), which is compared with a normal node. The severity of clinical infection varies considerably. The cardiac changes (**674**) are particularly severe, frequently leading to fatalities. The cause is a rickettsia-like organism, *Ehrlichia (Cytoecetes) ondiri*, which is present in circulating granulocytes and monocytes during the clinical syndrome, and later localises in the spleen and other organs. The disease is confined to altitudes above 1500 m in Kenya.

673

674

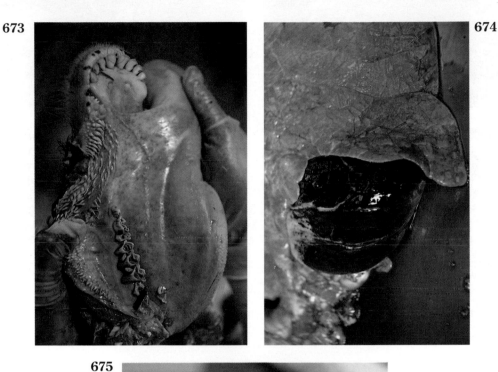

675

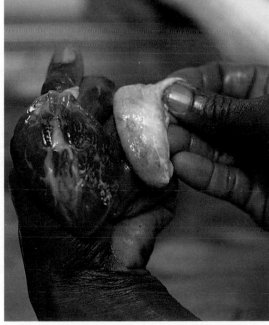

Jembrana disease

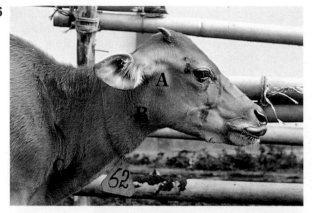

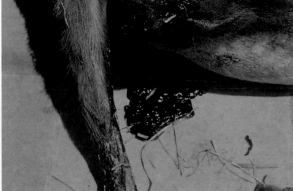

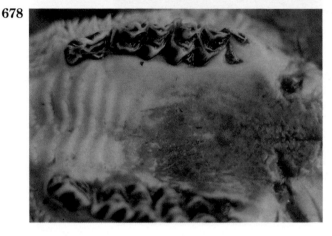

Characterised by a high mortality, and probably caused by an *Ehrlichia* carried by a *Boophilus* tick, Jembrana disease presents with clinical signs of pyrexia, marked lymphadenopathy (**676**), diarrhoes and haemorrhages. The cow (from Southern Africa) shows enlargement of the parotid (A), retropharyngeal (B) and prescapular nodes (C). The faeces may contain blood derived from intestinal mucosal haemorrhage (**677**). Postmortem examination reveals erosions on the hard and soft palates(**678**). *Differential diagnosis:* rinderpest (**634**).

Bali disease

Bali disease is a rickettsial limited to cattle on the Indonesian island of Bali. The characteristic sign is a peripheral necrosis of the ears (**679**), resulting from a generalised vasculitis. The clinical disease is probably related to Jembrana disease in Africa.

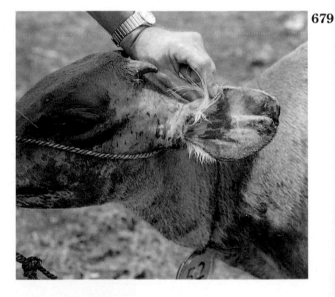

Trypanosomiasis

Of all animal diseases, the most important constraint on cattle production in the subhumid and humid tropics is trypanosomiasis, which in Africa alone affects animals in an area one third larger than the continental United States. Annual losses may be as high as US$50 billion. The disease also occurs in parts of Asia and in South America. A typical severely emaciated and anaemic N'Dama cow with *Trypanosoma vivax* infection in Mali is shown in **680**.

Since 1974, several major international efforts have been launched to control trypanosomiasis. Following unsuccessful attempts to use sterile male tsetse flies for breeding, as well as insecticides and chemotherapy, the tsetse fly control has concentrated on the installation of impregnated traps and screens. Furthermore, investigation of the phenomenon of trypanotolerance exhibited by several West and Central African cattle breeds, including the N'Dama, has been promising. The gross postmortem findings are variable and nonspecific, including enlargement of the lymph nodes and spleen (**681**), serous atrophy of fat, and anaemia. Confirmation depends on microscopic demonstration of trypanosomes in blood smears.

680

681

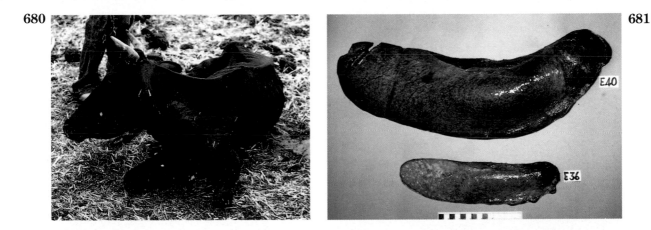

Bacterial diseases

Anthrax (splenic fever)

The characteristic feature of anthrax, seen clinically as sudden death in a previously healthy individual, is an enlarged, dark, soft-textured spleen, as seen in **682** in the specimen from a crossbred Hereford cow in Zimbabwe. The cause is *Bacillus anthracis*. Cattle suspected as possible anthrax cases should not undergo postmortem examination, and diagnosis should be based initially on a blood smear. Cattle may be infected through contaminated pastures (e.g., those flooded sporadically with river water carrying tannery effluent), or by eating contaminated artificial or natural feedstuffs. A vaccine is available.

682

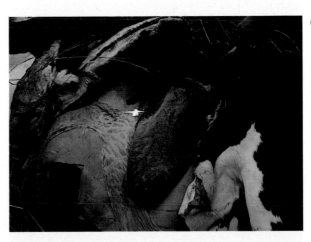

Clostridial diseases

Clostridia are natural inhabitants of the soil and of the gastrointestinal tract of man and animals. Pathogenic effects in cattle arise either from ingestion or from wound contamination. One group of clostridia produces disease by active invasion and toxin production leading to death (gas gangrene), the second produces toxins within the gut (enterotoxaemia), or in food or carrion outside the body (botulism). One clostridial disease, malignant oedema, is illustrated in the alimentary chapter (**165 & 166**) to aid in differential diagnosis from other conditions leading to swelling of the head. A range of combined clostridial vaccines is widely available and very effective in preventing disease.

Blackleg (*Clostridium chauvoei*)

Caused by *Cl. chauvoei*, blackleg develops spontaneously without a history of open wounds, although bruising may be a predisposing factor by producing anaerobic conditions in muscles that are harbouring the organism. Most cases end fatally after signs of acute depression and lameness. A carcase (**683**) may have extensive areas of darkened musculature. The hindquarters may have the most severe changes, including infiltration of the musculature with gas bubbles that have a characteristic rancid smell. Often, severely affected muscle (dark) lies adjacent to normal tissue (**684**). *Differential diagnosis*: malignant oedema (**166**).

683

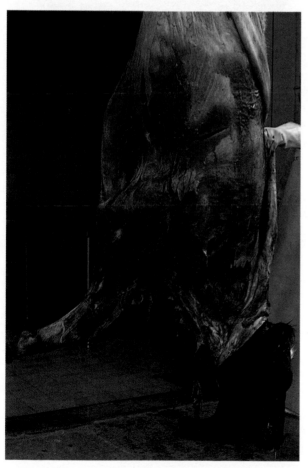

684

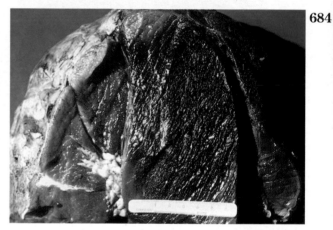

Tetanus *(Clostridium tetani,* 'lockjaw')

Introduced into deep, anaerobic skin wounds (e.g., castration, **526**), *Cl. tetani* causes progressive nervous signs as a result of neurotoxin production. Cattle show a generalised stiffness. The Jersey heifer in **685** has an extended head and neck, with the ears flattened back, and a raised tail. The nostrils may be dilated, and the third eyelid prolapsed. The disease progresses into severe extensor rigidity (**686**) with progressive respiratory failure. Note the severe opisthotonos. The rigidity is so severe that the upper feet remain off the ground. The tail is over-extended. The calf had been castrated two weeks previously. *Differential diagnosis* (in early cases): meningitis (**465**), cerebrocortical necrosis or polioencephalomalacia (**451**) hypomagnesaemic tetany in calves (**453**), and acute muscle dystrophy (**397**).

685
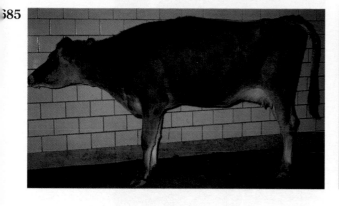

686
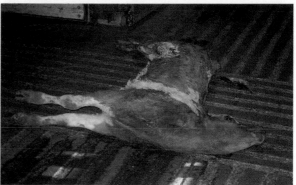

Botulism (*Clostridium botulinum*)

687
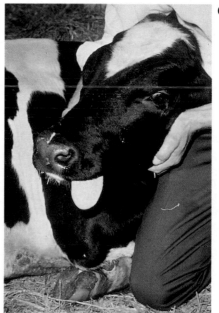

A rapidly fatal motor paralysis, caused by a *Cl. botulinum* neurotoxin (usually type D), results in initial posterior ataxia and progresses to paraparesis (**687**). The stance may be straddled (base-wide) and the hind fetlocks may be knuckled. Motor paralysis of the tongue (**688**) causes difficulty in prehension, chewing and swallowing. This cow could not hold its head up.

688

In **689** the Zebu cow had locomotor muscle weakness, paralysis of the head muscles and tongue prolapse. Other cows appear dull and may salivate profusely. Saliva may contain partially masticated feed material which cannot be swallowed (**690**). In some countries the major cause of botulism is the ingestion of decomposed animal carcases. This depraved appetite (pica) is stimulated by a phosphorus deficiency (**407 & 408**). Up to three per cent of cattle in endemic areas may die from botulism annually. Poultry litter utilised as cattle feed has also been implicated as a clostridial source. *Differential diagnosis*: organophosphorus toxicity (**723**), thromboembolic meningoencephalitis (**471**), BSE (**483**), SBE (**672**), and trauma.

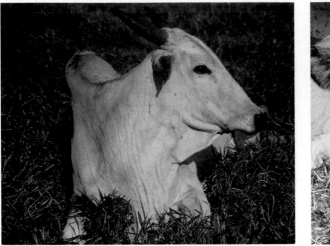

689

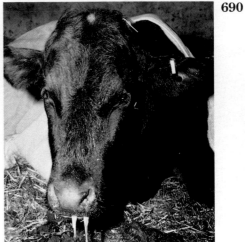

690

Miscellaneous

Bovine leukosis (bovine viral leukosis, bovine lymphosarcoma)

Leukosis occurs in four forms. The calfhood, thymic and skin types are all termed sporadic leukosis. The fourth type, the adult form, is known as enzootic bovine leukosis (EBL) and is caused by the bovine leukosis virus (BLV).

Calfhood multicentric lymphosarcoma

The calf in **691** showed generalised lymphadenopathy with gross enlargement of the prescapular node. The submandibular, parotid and retropharyngeal nodes were also symmetrically enlarged. Palpation revealed that the lymph nodes were smooth, painless and freely moveable, not involving the skin. Like other forms of bovine leukosis, calfhood leukosis has a low and sporadic incidence.

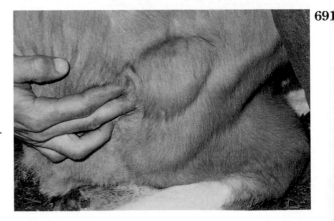

691

Thymic lymphosarcoma

A large, firm, smooth mass is present in the presternal region of the yearling Guernsey heifer in **692**. Oedema is also present. Most cases are seen in the 6–24 months age group. Generalised lymphadenopathy was absent. As in the multicentric form, a cross-section (**693**) of the discrete tumour from a 15-month-old crossbred Angus reveals pale yellow material without granulomatous contents.

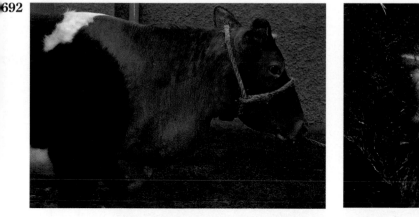

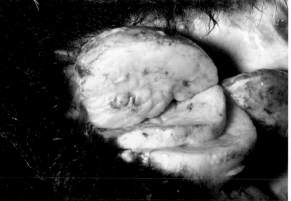

Skin lymphosarcoma

Skin leukosis is rare and is seen in immature animals aged 6–24 months. The crossbred Hereford in **694** has grey-white nodules over the neck, back and flanks, which extend deep into the subcutis. There is also a generalised lymphadenopathy with prominent precrural nodes. In **695** another animal has skin leukosis limited to large, ulcerated lesions around the head. *Differential diagnosis*: actinobacillosis (**161**), actinomycosis (**162**).

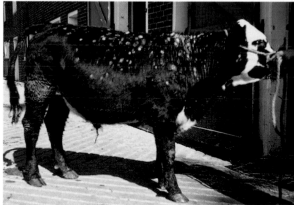

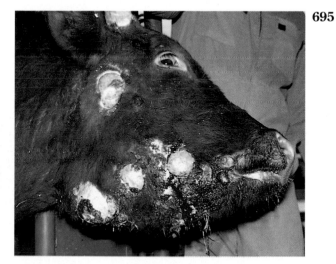

Enzootic (adult) bovine leukosis (EBL)

Enzootic bovine leukosis produces a generalised lymphadenopathy with symmetrical enlargement of most peripheral nodes, often with other signs. The Angus cow in **696** had enlarged submandibular, parotid (shaved for needle biopsy before photography) and prescapular nodes. Lymphosarcoma was also found in the heart and uterus. Some cases (20%) have a predilection, usually unilateral, for the orbit. The neoplasia is generally retrobulbar. Exceptionally, the adult cow in **697** has massive bilateral exophthalmos and protrusion of granulation tissue as a result of lymphomatous infiltration into the orbit. Other sites of lymphosarcoma include the globe itself (**449**), the spinal canal and cord, causing progressive posterior paresis as a result of spinal cord compression (**334**), and the abomasum (**196**).

696

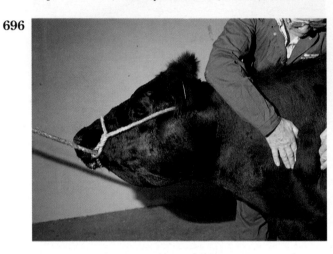

697

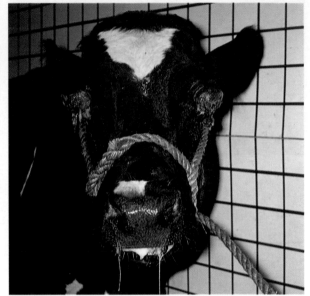

13 Toxicological disorders

Introduction

Illustrations of toxicological disorders in cattle present problems. The clinical signs may be transient, with death occuring within a few minutes, such as in yew (*Taxus baccata*) poisoning. In other cases, the signs may be nonspecific. Where the effects are confined largely to one system, the description has been given in the appropriate section, for example, ergot and fescue foot are dealt with under locomotor disorders (**401–403**). In this section, toxicoses have been broadly grouped into plant, organic and inorganic chemical sections.

Plant toxicoses

Bracken (bracken fern)

Bracken (*Pteridium aquilinum*) is usually a cumulative poison, acting in two ways. After ingesting large quantities for a few weeks, cattle may show an acute syndrome resulting from aplastic anaemia and thrombocytopenia. In **698** the vulva of the crossbred Angus cow is pale from severe anaemia. The pinpoint haemorrhages are a result of thrombocytopenia. Haemorrhages elsewhere can cause epistaxis, hyphaema (**699**) (bleeding into the anterior chamber) or haematuria from bladder mucosal haemorrhage (**700**).

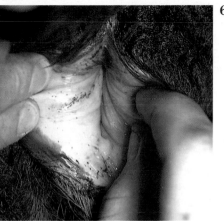
698

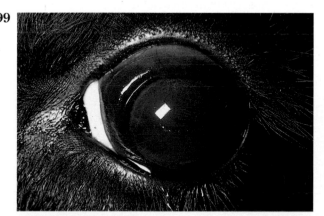
699

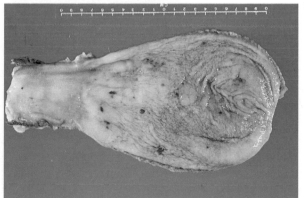
700

209

Ingestion of considerable quantities of bracken for several months can lead to a chronic syndrome. A carcinogen causes bladder neoplasia, resulting in enzootic haematuria and malignancies such as haemangiosarcoma (**701**). Numerous discrete masses are seen protruding from the mucosal surface. These bleed readily as the bladder distends and contracts. Some areas of mucosa (top right, lower left) appear normal. The haemangiomata can develop into ulcer-

ating tumours of various types. Alimentary tract neoplasms include squamous cell carcinomas and papillomas affecting the pharynx and oesophagus respectively. **702** shows pharyngeal squamous cell carcinomas (A) and oesophageal papillomas (B) from Brazil. Bracken toxicosis is widespread in several continents. A viral papilloma may be involved in upper alimentary neoplasms.

701

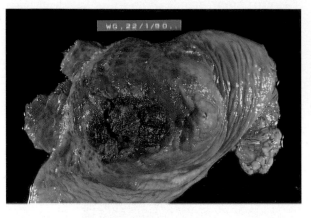

702

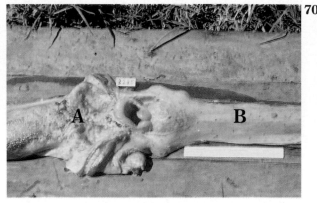

Oak (acorn)

Oak (*Quercus* species) may cause toxic signs following several days ingestion of acorns (autumn) or young leaves (spring). The toxic principle, a gallotannin, causes renal and gastrointestinal changes. The signs include abdominal pain, thirst, polyuria and ventral oedema as a result of subacute and chronic toxici-

ty. The oesophageal mucosa can be haemorrhagic (**703**). The enlarged swollen kidneys in **704** show scattered haemorrhages and a nephrosis, which accounts for the ventral oedema, ascites and hydrothorax seen in cases with renal failure.

703

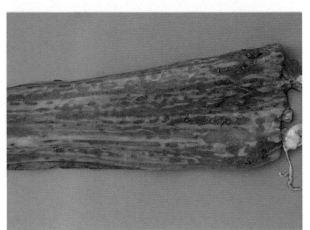

70

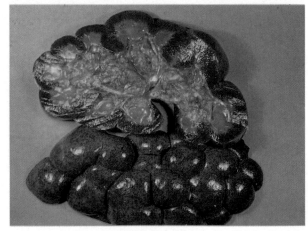

Yew

The opened rumen in **705** shows normal ingesta mixed with yew leaves. Yew (e.g., *Taxus baccata* – English yew, *T. cuspitata* – Japanese yew) contains a cardiotoxic alkaloid, taxine. Cattle usually die minutes after ingesting a few mouthfuls of yew twigs or berries, typically encountered as fresh or dried clippings thrown over a graveyard hedge into a bare winter pasture. The lethal dose in adult cattle may be as little as 1 kg of leaves.

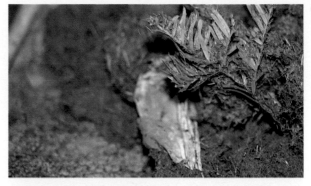
705

Ragwort

Ragwort (*Senecio jacobea*) contains a pyrrolizidine alkaloid, jacobine, that causes acute and chronic liver disease. Early signs include dark-coloured diarrhoea, photosensitisation, jaundice and central nervous system abnormalities. Prolonged ingestion results in liver failure due to cirrhosis, and severe lung disease. In the mature Hereford cow in **706**, the resulting right heart failure led to the ventral oedema affecting the ventral body wall, brisket and head.

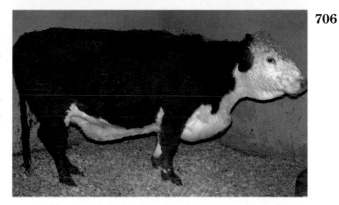
706

Rape and kale

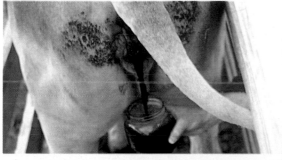
707

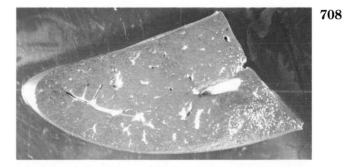
708

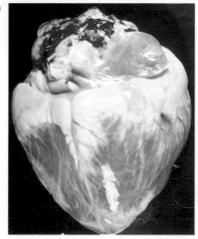
709

Some forms of forage of the *Brassica* family, such as kale and rape, contain S-methylcysteine sulphoxide, and can cause a haemolytic (Heinz body) anaemia following production of dimethyl disulphide by ruminal bacteria. Cattle develop haemoglobinuria, voiding dark-red urine (**707**), and are anaemic and weak. Postmortem examination of fatal cases reveals pallor and jaundice of the liver (**708**) and heart (**709**). *Differential diagnosis:* postparturient haemoglobinuria, bacillary haemoglobinuria (**213**), nitrate/nitrite poisoning (**724 & 725**), hypomagnesaemia (**454**), babesiosis (**655–660**), anaplasmosis (**661–664**) and acute bracken poisoning (**698–700**).

Lantana

Lantana camara is a shrub that causes hepatitis in cattle, producing signs of photosensitisation, jaundice, rumen stasis and depression. In **710** the Holstein steer from Zimbabwe shows severe skin lesions (typical of photosensitisation in that only the white areas are affected), depression, and tenesmus resulting from constipation. See also Chapter 3, photosensitisation p.30, and facial eczema p.214.

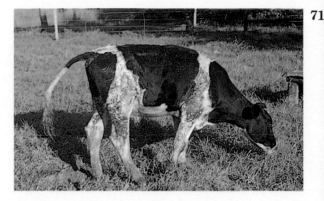

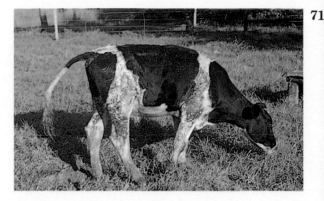 710

Solanum malacoxylon and *Trisetum flavescens* (enzootic calcinosis, enteque seco, espichamento)

In **711** the crossbred cow from Mato Grosso, Brazil is typically emaciated, stiff and stands on the toes of the forefeet. The endocardium and lungs of another cow (**712**) have areas of calcification (A), and the lungs have patches of ossified tissue (B). *Solanum malacoxylon* (South America) or *Trisetum flavescens* (Bavaria) acts by increasing calcium absorption from the gut through a metabolite of 1,25-dihydroxycholecalciferol, the active principle of vitamin D. It leads to excessive deposition of periosteal new bone and to calcifica-

tion of blood vessels, which may be appreciated on rectal palpation (aorta) and on the lower limb (distal arteries). Calcification of the deep flexor tendons and blood vessels is present in this German cow with *T. flavescens* toxicity in **713**. Other *Solanum* species cause cerebellar degeneration in Africa. The nightshade group (e.g., *Solanum negrum*, deadly nightshade) can produce gastrointestinal irritation and nervous signs.

711

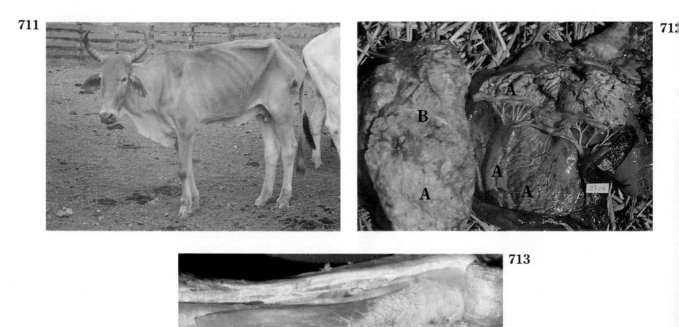

712

713

Tetrapterys species (*peito inchado*)

Tetrapterys species (*T. multiglandulosa* and *T. acutifolia*) cause a widespread cardiovascular disease in southeastern Brazil. Cattle develop ventral, especially brisket oedema (hence *peito inchado* or swollen breast), jugular venous distension and cardiac arhythmia, as seen in the five-year-old crossbred Zebu cow in **714**). The disease, usually subacute, is sometimes chronic, but rarely peracute. Postmortem lesions include myocardial pallor with some whitish streaking, and increased firmness suggestive of fibrosis, as seen in another mature Zebu cow in **715**. *Tetrapterys* poisoning has been reproduced by feeding fresh or dry plant material for 9–50 days. The same plant may be responsible for stillbirths.

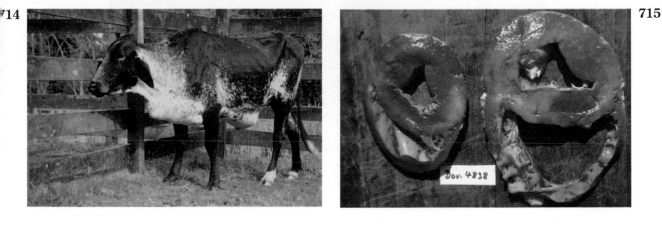

Selenium toxicity (locoweed, selenosis)

In **716** the extremely emaciated cow has extensive hair loss over the trunk, and claw deformities, resulting from prolonged ingestion of excessive selenium incorporated in *Astragalus* species, which are selenium accumulator plants. A horizontal band starts below the coronary band and moves slowly distally. Pain, producing severe lameness, results from the movement of wall horn over the exposed sensitive laminae (**717**). Affected cattle may be forced to graze in a kneeling position. Other toxins can also contribute to the clinical picture.

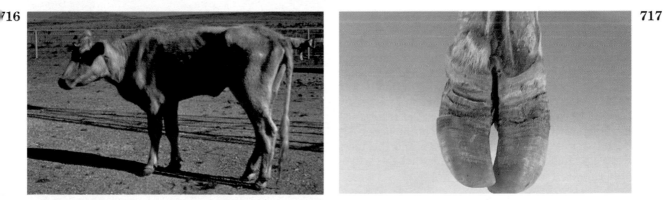

Lupine toxicity (crooked calf disease)

Deformed calves, with variable degrees of malalignment of the long bones, are born to cows that have ingested large quantities of certain species of lupine plants (e.g., *Lupinus caudatus*) during pregnancy. The calves in **718** were born to cows fed lupines from the fortieth to the seventieth day of gestation. Lupine species can also cause liver toxicity. See Chapter 1 (**12**) for other forms of arthrogryposis (e.g., BVD/MD virus infection).

718

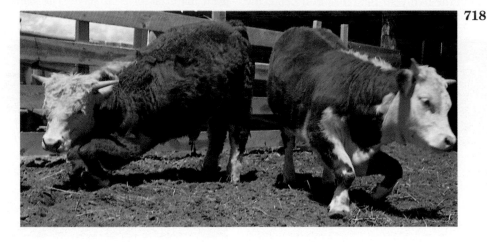

Mycotoxicoses

Mycotoxicosis is a poisoning due to the ingestion of a fungal toxin. One or more systems may be affected, but the photodermatitis associated with the fungus *Pithomyces chartarum* is the selected example.

Facial eczema

In facial eczema, an important disease in New Zealand, but also seen to a limited extent elsewhere, the fungus *Pithomyces chartarum* produces a hepatotoxic agent, sporidesmin. The fungus is commonly associated with ryegrass pastures. The clinical signs include lethargy, anorexia, jaundice and a photosensitive dermatitis. At an early stage, the thin skin of the udder of the Jersey cow in **719** had lost its hair, and a moist dermatitis and hyperaemia were evident. The skin in the upper left denuded area was starting to slough and the teats were also involved. Affected cows may lick this area of mild chronic irritation.

719

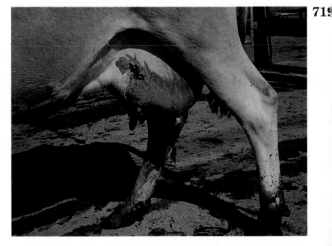

A late stage of facial eczema (720) shows a Friesian heifer with an extensive skin slough, typically confined to the white areas. Note the involvement of the forelimbs (A), where carpal flexion has caused sloughing, and the thickened, wrinkled appearance of the skin extending down the hind legs (B). In a Brazilian Zebu herd, a one-month-old male calf (721) had an extensive photodermatitis involving the ventral neck fold and chest wall and flank. The same fungus, *Pitho-* *myces chartarum*, was consumed by the dam from a pasture of *Brachiaria decubens*, sporidesmin being ingested through the milk. *Differential diagnosis*: other forms of photodermatitis.

Other examples of mycotoxicosis are illustrated in the locomotor section (fescue foot, **401**; ergot, **402** & **403**).Photosensitisation is covered in Chapter 3 (**70–75**).

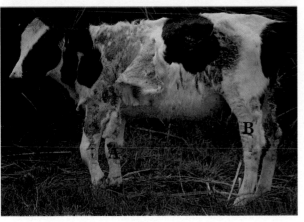

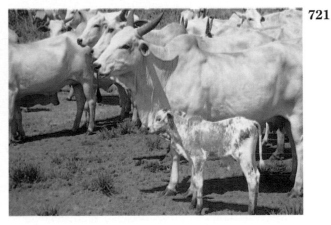

Organic toxicoses

Chlorinated naphthalenes

Naphthalenes were formerly extensively used as lubricants and wood-preserving compounds. They are compounds that cause hypovitaminosis A by interfering with the conversion of carotene to vitamin A. Hyperkeratosis of skin, emaciation, and possibly death, result when they are ingested over a long period. In **722** the head of the South African Friesian cow shows thickening, scaliness and wrinkling of skin. The hindquarters also had severe changes over the gaskin, hock, and metatarsus.

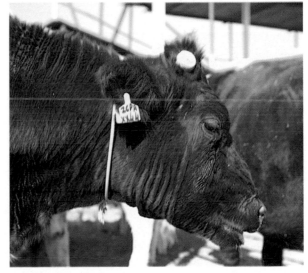

Carbamate and organophosphorus

Since the toxic signs of carbamate and organophosphorus tend to be similar, both of these organic groups can be discussed together.

The crossbred Angus cow in **723** had ingested a carbamate insecticide powder (carbofuran or 'Furadan') from a half-empty bag about 6–16 hours previously. Initial generalised muscle twitching, depression and locomotor incoordination were accompanied by hypersalivation. The cow then became semicomatose. Still salivating profusely, she showed miosis, severe dyspnoea and pronounced bradycardia, and died two hours later. The calf was healthy throughout. The clinical signs relate to the accumulation of acetylcho-

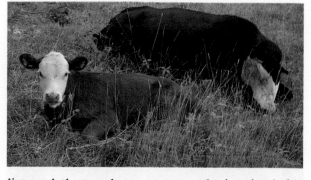

723

line and the resultant parasympathetic stimulation. *Differential diagnosis*: nitrate and cyanide poisoning (**724**), acute grain overload (**175**) and urea toxicity.

Inorganic chemical toxicoses

Nitrate/nitrite

Nitrates form nitrites before or after ingestion and cause respiratory distress because methaemoglobin formation leads to an anoxic anaemia. The sources of nitrate/nitrite are numerous and variable in type, and include cereals, specific plants, and both organic and inorganic fertilisers. A characteristic feature of this type of poisoning is the colour change in the vaginal mucosa. Levels of 22% (**724**) and 60% (**725**) met haemoglobin are illustrated. Clinical signs appear at a level of about 20% conversion of haemoglobin to methaemoglobin, while death follows at 60–80%. *Differential diagnosis*: silo gas poisoning, sodium chlorate poisoning, acute rape or kale toxicity (**707**), and cyanide, carbon dioxide, cobalt or chronic copper poisoning(**729**).

724

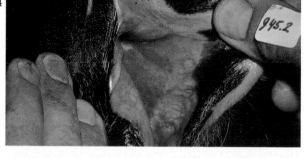

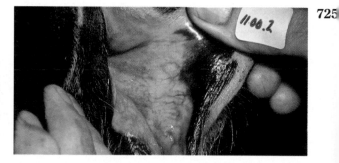725

Lead

In lead poisoning the major signs of central nervous system (CNS) involvement are depression, blindness and, often, head-pressing. The one-month-old Gloucester calf in **726** shows severe CNS signs. Unable to stand, its head and neck are extended to push against the brick wall. It was also blind and anorexic. Lead is a common toxicological problem in younger cattle. The source is often paint from old doors, as in this calf, although crankcase oil from farm machinery, lead batteries, contaminated feedstuffs and golf balls are other sources. *Differential diagnosis:* polioencephalomalacia (CCN) (**451**), listeriosis (**459**) and meningitis (**465**).

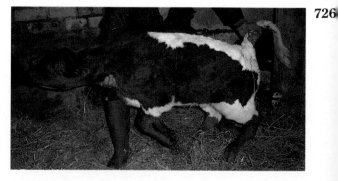726

Fluorosis

Fluorosis usually results from the prolonged ingestion of fluorine in high fluorine-phosphatic supplementary feeds, or from herbage ingested from pastures contaminated by industrial emissions. Large periosteal plaques form on long bones. **727** shows several enlargements that are firm and smooth to the touch on the medial aspects of the metatarsi. In **728** the extensive periosteal plaques, which do not involve the artic-

ular surfaces, are seen next to normal metatarsi (to the left). Cattle may become lame owing to osteoporosis and periarticular bone proliferation. Another sign of chronic disease is mottling of the temporary incisors (see **154**). *Differential diagnosis:* degenerative joint disease (**361**), aphosphorosis (**407**) and selenosis (**716**).

727

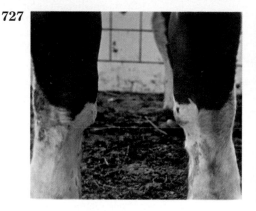

728

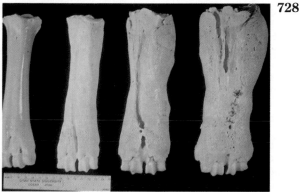

Copper

Copper toxicosis in cattle tends to be chronic, although the onset of clinical signs may be acute and associated with stress. The source may be an error of copper supplementation, or ingestion of pasture with an abnormal level of copper (from slurry or fertiliser top-dressing) . Affected animals have dark urine due to haemoglobinuria. The major postmortem changes include a large, friable, icteric liver and a characteristic bluish-black ('gunmetal') colouring of the kidneys (**729**).

729

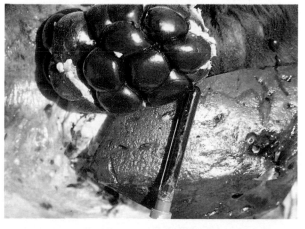

Molybdenum

Molybdenum toxicosis tends to involve a relative copper deficiency. The cow from China (**730**) is thin and shows depigmentation of the normally dark coat. Note the greyish hairs around the eyes. Alopecia is present over the neck, shoulder and withers. Note the combination halter and nose-ring used in Jiangxi Province. Many cattle with molybdenum toxicity show a persistent diarrhoea. This is typical of the high-molybdenum 'teart' pastures in parts of England. Cattle respond to copper supplementation. *Differential diagnosis:* copper deficiency (**410**) and cobalt deficiency (**416**).

730

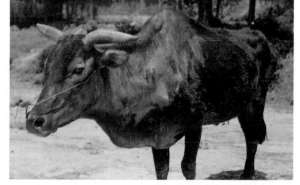

INDEX

Figures refer to page numbers